Clinical Audit for Doctors

Margaret G Keane
Chen Sheng Low
Bhoresh Dhamija

Edited by Robert Ghosh

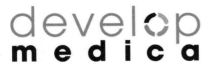

Published by Developmedica 2009
Castle Court
Duke Street
New Basford,
Nottingham, NG7 7JN
0845 838 0571
www.developmedica.com

Developmedica recommends that you consult your hospital's Audit department, the National Institute for Health and Clinical Excellence (NICE) and the NHS Executive web sites for information and guidance relating to the understanding and undertaking of Clinical Audit. The views expressed in this book are those of Developmedica and not those of the National Health Service. Developmedica is in no way associated with the National Health Service or NICE.

The contents of this book are intended as a guide only and although every effort has been made to ensure that the contents of this book are correct, Developmedica cannot be held responsible for the outcome of any loss or damage that results from the use of this guide. Readers are advised to seek independent advice regarding the understanding of Clinical Audit together with consulting the institution for which the audit is performed.

Every effort has been made to contact the copyright holders of any material reproduced within this publication. If any have been inadvertently overlooked, the publishers will be pleased to make restitution at the earliest opportunity.

A catalogue record for this title is available from the British Library.

ISBN 978-1-9068390-1-7

Typeset by Replika Press Pvt. Ltd. (India)

Printed by Bell & Bain Ltd., Glasgow

1 2 3 4 5 6 7 8 9 10

Mixed Sources
Product group from well-managed forests and other controlled sources
www.fsc.org   Cert no. TT-COC-002769
© 1996 Forest Stewardship Council
FSC

Contents

About the editor

Robert Ghosh

Robert Ghosh is a Consultant Physician at Homerton University Hospital, London. He is the Director of Intensive Care and Director of Acute Medicine.

As Trust Lead for Clinical Audit and Chair of the Clinical Audit and Effectiveness Committee, he has facilitated robust relationships between key committees in order to feed into the Clinical Audit system. He has thereby implemented strategic innovations which have allowed operational issues such as risk and complaints to develop into vehicles for quality, through clinical audit.

About the authors

Margaret G Keane

Margaret G Keane MBBS BSc AKC MRCP is an ITU 'Specialist Trainee 1' at the Hammersmith Hospital in London. She trained at Guys, Kings and St Thomas Medical School. Margaret has undertaken periods of research at Kings College London and Johns Hopkins University Baltimore. She has had a long-standing interest and involvement in clinical audit, having completed more than 20 audit projects largely in topics related to intensive care and gastrointestinal pathology.

Chen Sheng Low

Chen Sheng Low Adv. Dip. in Medical Sciences MBChB MRCP (London) MRCP (Edin) is a Specialist Registrar in Nuclear Medicine in the West Midlands Deanery based at City Hospital, Birmingham. He trained at the University of Aberdeen. He has conducted numerous clinical audits, and has presented in national and international conferences. He is also currently a Clinical Tutor for medical students, whom he oversees in their own clinical audit projects. His other interests include the delivery of courses on how to do well at interview. He has a thorough understanding of the importance of clinical audit for doctors.

Bhoresh Dhamija

Bhoresh Dhamija is a neurosurgical trainee working in the West Midlands Deanery, based at the Queen Elizabeth Hospital, Birmingham. Following undergraduate studies at St.Andrews University (BSc in Medical science) and Manchester University

(MBChB), he worked as a Demonstrator in Anatomy at Cambridge University, teaching undergraduate students a Regional based anatomy syllabus. On completion of the primary MRCS Bhoresh moved on to a Basic Surgical Rotation with the Hammersmith Hospitals. He has participated and presented at several national and international neurosurgical conferences and published articles in established surgical journals.

About the publisher

Developmedica is a specialist provider of books, courses and eLearning solutions tailored to meet your career development needs. Visit our web site at www.developmedica.com and find out more.

Our approach is friendly and personal. Please telephone or email any time to discuss your requirements.

Free companion material available from the Developmedica web site

If you are planning or conducting a clinical audit, you will need to register your audit, collect data and document actions. A number of resources illustrated in this book will assist you.

Working pro formas of these illustrations, which you may take and adapt to your own purposes, can be downloaded free of charge from the Developmedica web site at www.developmedica.com.

Acknowledgements

For my niece Abigail Cohen, whose life was short but wide.
Robert Ghosh

I would like to thank Ted Keane for his continued support.
Margaret Geraldine Keane

I would like to thank Dr. Alp Notghi, Consultant Physician in Nuclear Medicine, City Hospital for all his help and support.
Chen Sheng Low

For Mum and Dad for their continued wisdom, help and support.
Bhoresh Dhamija

We would all like to thank Matt Green, Sarah Silvester and Jen Neal for all their support during the writing of this book.

Margaret Geraldine Keane, Chen Sheng Low and Bhoresh Dhamija

Foreword

Over the last half century, wider use of clinical evidence has transformed patient outcomes. However, the potential of medical advances to improve the quality of patient care has not fully been realised. Many barriers exist to the implementation of best practice. Through careful analysis of healthcare delivery, these barriers can be recognised and overcome. Since the publication of *Working for Patients* in 1989, clinical audit has evolved from an abstract concept to a core part of professional practice.

Audit is a valuable tool to drive quality improvement and decrease the variation between organisations' performance against quality criteria. The process of examining current practice, then making changes and looking for evidence of improvement, is at the heart of this. Done frequently and well, clinical audit has the potential to transform services for patients, resulting in a significant positive shift in the quality of health organisations. To deliver excellent care, we must guard against audit becoming simply an obligation to progress through training or satisfy clinical governance boards.

High Quality Care For All (2008) highlights the need to increase clinical involvement in NHS leadership and management. Clinical audit empowers those who deliver care to improve the service in which they work. Data can and should be harnessed locally to help doctors deliver care that is consistently effective, safe and acceptable to patients. Beacons of excellence can influence policy on a local, regional and national level and so lead to service improvement throughout the NHS. In this way, today's doctors are given the opportunity to develop into tomorrow's clinical leaders.

As NHS resources are stretched by the needs of an ageing population and the costs of technological advances, refinements in healthcare delivery will become central to maintaining high quality service provision. This book provides practical advice on performing rigorous and effective clinical audit and I am convinced that audit will prove invaluable in ensuring that we deliver excellent and high value clinical services. It is our professional responsibility to ensure that we use these tools to continue to shift the mean of the quality curve for clinical performance.

Sir Liam Donaldson
Chief Medical Officer (England)
Department of Health

Preface

Clinical audit, the tool for quality

Since at least the 1980s, movers and shakers in healthcare politics have reiterated two core desires. Firstly, doctors should be firmly entrenched in process changes which improve quality of care. Secondly, clinical audit should be a fundamental model of just such a process. These themes were prominent in the Griffiths report in 1983, *Working for Patients* in 1989, the NHS Plan in 2000 and more recently in the Tooke and Darzi reports. Drivers for progressing clinical audit have also been prominent within the radar of the Care Quality Commission (CQC), General Medical Council (GMC) and the Postgraduate Medical Education and Training Board (PMETB).

In recent years clinicians have been absorbed in pursing nationally driven 'targets', which many have found simultaneously all-consuming and grudgingly relevant. The old adage of 'if you meet your target, you will achieve quality' has been innovatively inverted by the wise and the good to 'if you achieve quality, your target will be easier to attain'. If we are indeed emerging into a brave new healthcare world focussed on quality, this debate fits wholesale within the realms of clinical audit. Acute and other trusts need to pay more than lip service to the fact that clinical audit is an itemised core standard. They will have to demonstrate to the CQC that they are measuring their criteria and their standards, and that they are translating clinical audit outcomes into action, and action into improved quality. Educational and process strategies need to be factored into reports, as does evidence that time and funding constraints are considered by the trust. Although these requirements by the CQC (like any other CQC requirement) may generate temporary anxiety, individuals are finally getting the message that improved quality is the objective. Although it seems intuitive that many efficiency strategies may lead to cost savings for institutions such as acute trusts, realistically some quality drives may lead to increased expenditure; this may make healthcare management challenging, with an ongoing economic recession at the time of writing.

The fact that the GMC and PMETB refuse to see clinical audit as a tick-box exercise should alert and interest all doctors, including appraisers. The topic should not be sidestepped or dismissed by the appraisee, nor should it be allowed to by the appraiser. Relevance, detail and evidence of quality assurance should be sought. In the near future, this will also be relevant for re-validation.

The fact that this book is titled 'Clinical Audit *for Doctors*' may seem perverse when most clinical governance forums advocate a multidisciplinary approach. My intention, though agreeing wholeheartedly with the multidisciplinary sentiment, was blatant. I was tired of witnessing the lack of clinical audit books in the medical section of bookshops, and wanted to engage the widest spectrum of doctors. I would wish to clarify slightly oxymoronically that although this book is particularly for doctors, it is also relevant for any budding clinical auditor.

Doctors Dhamija, Keane and Low, all trainee doctors, have done admirably in contributing to factual and punchy chapters which will be relevant to the whole spectrum of the medical profession. Established consultants and all junior doctors, from Foundation doctors to specialist trainees, should find this book a useful reference both for mentorship and for devising new projects. Medical students, who are increasingly in tune with the benefits of clinical audit, may also benefit.

The book deals with, among other things, issues relating to history and definition, identification of criteria and standards, the role of the clinical audit department, data analysis and interpretation, presentation, implementation and re-audit. Many useful pointers are given to assist with involvement in clinical audit and the construction of a successful project.

I sincerely hope that you find this book relevant, useful and rewarding.

Happy auditing.

Robert Ghosh

Chapter 1 Clinical audit: history and definition

What is clinical audit?

Clinical audit is the process of evaluating clinical practice against adopted guidelines, implementing necessary changes into clinical practice and subsequently reassessing the difference that these changes have made. The overall objective of this process is to ensure high standards of clinical practice and to improve the overall quality of patient care. Clinical audit has been defined by the National Institute for Health and Clinical Excellence in their 2002 document *Principles for Best Practice in Clinical Audit* as:

> 'A quality improvement process that seeks to improve patient care and outcomes through systematic review of care against explicit criteria and the review of change. Aspects of the structure, process and outcome of care are selected and systematically evaluated against explicit criteria. Where indicated changes are implemented at an individual, team, or service level further monitoring is used to confirm improvement in healthcare delivery.'

The Department of Health (DH) defined clinical audit succinctly in their 1989 White Paper *Working for Patients* as:

> 'The systematic critical analysis of the quality of medical care including the procedures used for diagnosis and treatment, the use of resources and the resulting outcome and quality of life for the patient.'

Where did clinical audit begin?

Between 1853 and 1855 Florence Nightingale nursed soldiers from the Crimean war in a hospital in the medical barracks in Scutari. She observed the high mortality rates among patients and believed them to be related to the unsanitary conditions within the camp. Noting this trend, Nightingale instigated a change in practice among her team of 38 nursing staff. She introduced strict sanitary routines and standards of hygiene to the hospital and equipment. After these changes she collected detailed records of mortality among the hospital patients, and identified two groups that were as uniform as possible, with the only change being hygiene management. The mortality rate in the group where strict hygiene was practised was 2 per cent compared with 40 per cent in the standard group. Immediately, doctors and officers with the British army could see the benefit of these changes and embraced them as part of routine practice. Although this study mainly embraced the criteria of clinical research (scientific evaluation of best practice), it heralded the concept of standards.

Ernest Codman (1869–1940) was a surgeon working in Massachusetts. He carefully followed up each of his surgical patients to identify any short- and long-term complications of the operations. This use of process is very familiar to any surgical department today and is usually the focus of their regular audit meetings. Although it is not commonplace to compare complication rates nationally and internationally by validated audited data, this concept was revolutionary at the time, though not widely adopted.

Despite the successes of Florence Nightingale in the Crimea, the growth of clinical audit was slow over the next century, with the process being adopted only occasionally by healthcare professionals to evaluate the quality of the healthcare that they provided.

This changed significantly in 1983, when the Health Secretary Norman Fowler instituted an enquiry into the effective use of manpower in the NHS. The subsequent report was led by Roy Griffiths, the Deputy Chairman and Managing Director of Sainsburys. The response to the finding of the lack of coherent management at the local (hospital) level led to some key recommendations, including the commencement of clinical audit.

In 1989 improving healthcare had become a hot political issue, and had to be addressed by Margaret Thatcher's Government. The Department of Health produced a white Paper, *Working for Patients*. This introduced the concept of the 'internal market' where funding components were itemised, often via complex contractual processes, while preserving the concept of healthcare remaining 'free at the point of delivery'. Clinical audit was absolutely fundamental to the key philosophy of maintaining quality in the face of budgeting.

By the early 1990s, clinical audit had become mandatory for clinicians and participation was itemised in many of their contracts. As the number of clinical audits being undertaken in trusts grew substantially, increasingly more members of the multidisciplinary team became involved.

Subsequent to the change in government in 1997 and the introduction of the 'NHS Plan' by the New Labour government, several separate additional approaches to improve quality in the NHS were introduced. Clinicians were encouraged to engage in clinical audit, and it was recognised that the latter could be a potent vehicle for achieving clinical effectiveness (Donaldson and Gray 1998). There was also a move to improve organisational quality through initiatives such as the Patients' Charter, and reducing waiting lists and waiting times. Patient empowerment was enhanced, through analysis of patient satisfaction (via patient satisfaction surveys) and novel complaints systems.

These days, well-publicised scandals and the growth in evidenced-based medicine have changed the way that healthcare is practised by doctors and other healthcare professionals. There is rightly an emphasis on increasingly patient-centred care. With the expansion of the internet, health information is more readily available and patients are therefore much more informed. Clinical audit has become an increasingly important tool to measure our practice in a transparent way and assess the overall quality of the service provided. Healthcare modernisation has allowed clinical audit to adopt a very high profile, and become ingrained in healthcare practice for the future.

The position of clinical audit within clinical governance

The concept of clinical governance has been transferred from the commercial sector. In 1992, a number of incidents led the government to recommend standards for financial management to companies in the private sector for adopting new rules on accountability and conduct. These ideas were transferred to healthcare, with clinical governance becoming a requirement for the NHS (Committee on Standards in Public Life 1995). Clinical governance was (and still is) defined as:

'A framework through which NHS organisations are accountable for continuously improving the quality of their services and safeguarding high standards of care by creating an environment in which excellence in clinical care will flourish.' (Scally & Donaldson, 1998).

Initially, six facets of clinical governance were identified, including clinical audit. The other five were education and training, clinical effectiveness, research and development, openness and risk management. These components still make up the core of most clinical governance meetings today. However, categorising and isolating a set number of elements is now considered too simplistic, and probably carries a risk of ignoring other key components. All activities leading to the maintenance and improvement of clinical excellence should be within the remit of clinical governance.

In the 1990's chief executives of NHS trusts and primary care trusts for the first time became directly accountable for the quality of service provided by their organisations. From April 1999, acute and community NHS trusts had developed established structures and processes for effective clinical governance. The implementation and development of clinical governance are continuing to be regularly monitored by the Care Quality Commission.

It is important to recognise some overarching principles within clinical governance: clear lines of responsibility and acceptability for the overall quality of clinical care; a comprehensive programme of quality improvement activities – including clinical audit; clear policies aimed at managing risks; and procedures for all professional groups to identify and remedy poor performance.

The audit cycle

Clinical audit is a process with five main parts that is commonly described as the audit cycle (Figure 1.1). Once the area or standard for audit is defined, the journey around the cycle perpetuates, with the completing of 'the loop' leading to the commencement of another

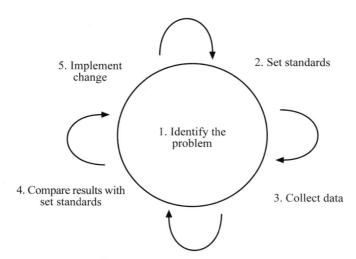

Figure 1.1   The audit cycle.

cycle, and another chapter in the drive for improved quality. One good result from clinical audit does not imply everlasting success.

Stage 1: Identification of the problem

Before embarking on an audit it is important to outline the topic carefully. The plans should be discussed with all the relevant members of the team. At this stage it is important to outline any national or local standards or guidelines that exist and undertake a literature search in order to acquire a thorough understanding of the problem.

Stage 2: Definition of criteria and standards

The aim of the audit, and the data and information needed, should be identified by the team. The criteria are explicit statements that define the activity that is being measured, and represent elements of care that may be measured objectively.

The identification of criteria should lead to the definition of the standards for comparison. This may be a local hospital or national guideline that has been validated and is widely available in most areas of clinical practice. The chosen guideline should be up-to-date and represent a summary of the best evidence for clinical practice. When guidelines do not exist, other standards may be considered – this may include self-constructed standards in the absence of a pre-defined guideline. One may use the results of another group as a standard; however for this to be valid it is important that this group is selected carefully in order to avoid biasing the audit.

Stage 3: Data collection

Data collection is time-consuming and may be the most recognisable part of audit for many. The data should be collected as accurately and efficiently as possible; this should be methodical and precise, and the methodology should be similar for each patient. It may be prudent to try to collect more data than initially calculated, as revisiting data collection is tedious and time-consuming. The populations and exceptions should be clearly defined. The study period should also be defined very clearly (e.g. 'all admissions to a surgical ward over a 28-day period'). All data should be anonymised and stored according to national and local data handling guidelines. The sample size is important: the larger the size, the greater the statistical validity of the results.

Stage 4: Comparison of performance with standard, and presentation

The next stage involves careful compilation of the collected data, looking for trends and differences. The results are subsequently analysed and compared with the standard identified. If standards were not adhered to, it is important to attempt to identify the reasons for this together with suggestions for improvement. The presentation should be to your relevant department, and also all relevant members of healthcare personnel. This usually implies a wide audience. Here, critical discussion and implementation plans should be facilitated.

Stage 5: Implementing change

This is often the most difficult, vital and ignored stage of the audit process. A great deal of work has gone in to the previous stages, in order to demonstrate findings. It is therefore important that changes are initiated, the cycle completed and improvement implemented. Hopefully action plans and key individuals are at least briefly described at the end of the presentation.

It may be relevant on occasions to recommend changes to a guideline or the implementation of a new guideline. This is a very important step in order to standardise practice and improve quality. However, guidelines take a long time to be approved, as they pass though various committees. It is therefore important that this part of the process is undertaken by someone who will be in the department for long enough to see the process through.

Re-audit

This forms the final part of the audit process – the 'closure of the loop'. The length of time to re-audit may be variable; however every effort should be made to suggest a date when plans are made for implementation (see above). The date set should be realistic, and allow for the implementation plans to be achieved. The criteria in re-audit should ideally be exactly similar to those in the original audit.

These stages reinforce the values of perpetual movement and improvement, particularly with regard to analysing personal practice, implementing change and improving the overall quality of healthcare.

Triggers for projects

It is vital to identify a trigger, as the latter will help concentrate the mind, and also itemise the drivers for clinical effectiveness. Examples include:

- Perception – the perceived notion that an activity needs to be audited (either because it is performed badly or well.)

- Adverse event – an incident or series of incidences.

- Patient Outcome Monitoring – this will include formal complaints, patients' experiences and patients' perceived outcome.

- National guideline – it is good practice to assess national standards on a rolling programme. Although many national guidelines may not be mandatory, Trusts must show they capture and assess every item in a certain category (e.g. NICE guidelines) and define relevance and appropriateness. If the guideline is relevant and appropriate, it would be prudent to audit against it.

- National diktat – a mandatory audit from a national authoritative body (e.g. NPSA, Department of Health, Care Quality Commission.)

- Local Guideline – it is good practice to audit against local standards on a rolling programme.

- Local diktat – the Trust attaches importance to a national guideline or local guideline, and makes an audit mandatory.

- Triggers will be dealt with in greater detail in Chapter 4 of this book.

Doctors and other healthcare professionals: roles and barriers

Clinical audit is a core example of a topic where multi-disciplinary and multi-professional team working is vital. The various roles, from lead auditing to data handling and presentation, should be adopted by those most dedicated and able.

Most healthcare professionals have been exposed to clinical audit and generally have an appreciation of the process and purpose of audit. Although there is occasional scepticism and resistance to participation, there is evolving evidence that where audit loops have been closed there has been an overall improvement in patient care (Gabbay *et al.*, 1990). It is important to set aside any scepticism, and recognise clinical audit as a tool to improve the quality of healthcare.

Barriers to embarking on a clinical audit project, such as busy lives, significant on-call commitments, high patient loads, operating lists and outpatient clinics are regularly encountered. Many projects remain unfinished. Furthermore, it is not uncommon for results of audits not to lead to implementation plans and a relevant change in practice. It is therefore not surprising that healthcare providers become discouraged and question the value of the clinical audit process. It is vital, therefore, that the importance and role of clinical audit is perpetually reinforced, and that the whole process is supported and overseen.

Completing a whole audit cycle is not a short process. Junior doctors may change jobs every 2–3 months, and as a result it may be difficult to complete a whole audit in one job. Hence it is important to try to get involved in different parts of the audit process in each new job. Involvement is the key, rather than the specific commencement or presentation of a project. This will enable individuals to contribute to more projects while in short-term posts, and also develop an awareness of issues in the whole cycle. Hospital trusts need to buy into this process by recognising the contribution of junior doctors, even when they have rotated on to another post.

Clinical audit as a process of improving patient care works best when the idea for the audit comes from those with most clinical contact. They are usually best able to observe difficulties in practice, trends and problems with guidelines and practice. The discussion of clinical problems within multidisciplinary teams should be encouraged. The translation of this discussion into an audit project should also remain multidisciplinary. This will hopefully ensure team working, and perhaps wider implementation of any findings.

The involvement of national bodies

Increasingly professional bodies including Royal Colleges, Deaneries and Foundation schools all now actively support clinical audit, and often run large audits in which they encourage trainees to participate.

Medical training in the UK also now demands that doctors understand clinical audit and participate in the process.

The Royal College of Physicians (RCP, www.rcplondon.ac.uk) and Royal College of Surgeons (RCS, 2000) have both advocated the role of clinical audit within clinical practice.

The Department of Health have established various forums including the National Clinical Audit and Patients' Outcomes Programme (NCAPOP) and Healthcare Quality Improvement Partnership (HQIP). The latter body has expanded from simply commissioning clinical audits to facilitating service improvement. This remit will include a role in supporting the newly created National Clinical Audit Advisory Group (NCAAG), which was set up to provide advice and guidance on the overall programme of work, in particular to consider proposals for new audits or for discontinuing existing audits. In addition they will have responsibility for reinvigorating both national and local clinical audit, bringing together clinicians and other stakeholders to ensure that clinical audit takes its rightful place as a key mechanism for improving service quality. The NCAAG activities will include advising the Department of Health on matters relating to NCAPOP.

For further detail, see the section in Chapter 2 on national bodies and national clinical audits.

Clinical audit and interviews

Every interview application form, ranging from Foundation to Consultant posts, requests details of clinical audit experience. Within these questions the assessors are looking for a candidate to show an appreciation of the value of clinical audit, an understanding of the audit process (including implementation and re-audit), the interpretation of findings and the ability to describe involvement. By conducting an audit doctors are showing commitment; the process of collecting data usually takes weeks to months and requires the highest standard of organisation and time management. Communication skills are often tested, as explanations to patients may be required in order to address any questions or concerns that they have. The collation and scrutiny of data demonstrates an understanding of statistical analysis. Presentation of your results and findings demonstrates your ability to deliver a lecture and discuss data coherently with your peers. Involvement in implementation and plans for re-audit implies an interest in the whole process of change, including education.

Candidates are often asked to discuss their best or most recent audit, or to discuss an audit where the loop has, or has not, been closed. Here, the panel is often seeking an awareness of the validity of standards, the difficulties in implementation and demonstration of genuine involvement.

Clinical audit and appraisal

Trainees and Consultants are appraised at least annually, and occasionally more frequently. In appraisals it would be rare not to be asked about clinical audit. Increasingly, the questions asked will cease to be 'tick-box' in nature, and the answers will need to be accompanied by a discussion involving the detail of triggers, standards and implementation plans. Involvement may be demonstrated by the appraisee with the use of project reference numbers.

Guidelines and diktats from government bodies and from within the trust

Government bodies (for example the NPSA, Department of Health and Care Quality Commission) may issue diktats to trusts making certain audit projects mandatory. The occasional national guideline may emanate (for example from NICE) for consideration. It is good practice (and may become mandatory practice) to keep a log of all national guidelines and diktats. These may be identified by correspondence from the relevant body to the trust, or by active seeking by the Clinical Audit Department. Experts within the Trust should assess the relevance and appropriateness of the guideline and identify the nature of alternative guidelines (if appropriate). One may then embark upon a clinical audit project, using the relevant guideline as a standard.

Awareness of local guidelines will often serve as triggers for audit projects. Healthcare employers such as acute trusts may issue local diktats for audit, as particular importance may be attached to a national guideline or local guideline.

Some may take issue with the notion that clinicians and other individuals are 'instructed' to perform audit. This potential irritation should be superseded by the understanding that a robust process will facilitate forever improving clinical standards.

Key points

- Audit is 'the systematic critical analysis of the quality of medical care including the procedures used for diagnosis and treatment, the use of resources and the resulting outcome and quality of life for the patient' (DH 1989)

- Clinical audit has a pivotal role in clinical governance and appraisal

- Clinical audit is a perpetual spiral which provides continuous assessment of standards and improved quality of care. Implementation is key, as is re-audit

- Triggers for audits should be clearly defined; this will help concentrate the mind, and also itemise the drivers for clinical effectiveness

- It is important to have an awareness of diktats and guidelines issued by national bodies

References

Department of Health (1989) *Working for Patients: Medical Audit Working Paper No. 6.* HMSO, London. Paragraph 1.1.

Donaldson, L. & Gray, J. (1998) Clinical governance: a quality duty for health organisations. *Quality and Safety in Health Care*, 7 (suppl.), BMJ, London, S37–S44.

Gabbay J, McNicol MC, Spiby J, Davies SC, Layton AJ. (1990) What did audit achieve? Lessons from preliminary evaluation of a year's medical audit. *British Medical Journal*, Volume 301, pp. 526-529

Griffiths Report (1983), NHS Management Inquiry Report. DHSS, London.

NICE (2002). *Principles and Best Practice in Clinical Audit.* Radcliffe Medical Press Ltd., Oxford, page10.

RCS – Faculty of Dental Surgeons. 2000. Methodologies for Clinical Audit in Dentistry. See www.rcseng.ac.uk/fds/clinical guidelines.

RCP – See www.rcplondon.ac.uk/clinical-standards.

Scally G and Donaldson L.J., Clinical governance and the drive for quality improvement in the new NHS in England, *British Medical Journal,* (4 July 1998): 61–65.

Chapter 2   The pathway to clinical effectiveness

What is clinical effectiveness?

In the modern National Health Service (NHS), healthcare services have become increasingly regulated in order to try to maintain the highest standards, both operationally and clinically.

Clinical effectiveness can be defined as:

> 'The extent to which specific clinical interventions, when deployed in the field for a particular patient or population, do what they are intended to do, i.e. maintain and improve health and secure the greatest possible health gain from available resources' (NHS Executive 1996).

But perhaps the best definition of clinical effectiveness is as follows.

'The right person (healthcare professional) doing:

- The right thing (evidence-based practice)

- In the right way (skills and competence)

- At the right time (providing treatment/services in the appropriate time)

- In the right place (location of treatment/services)

- With the right result (maximising health gains)'

Therefore, clinical effectiveness motivates healthcare professionals to think constantly about applying the best evidence-based care for the best outcomes. Certainly, if any of the above criteria were to be compromised, a change in practice may need to be implemented. Clinical effectiveness is the aspiration at all levels of NHS provision from Strategic Health Authority (SHA), via the trust board, to the individual clinician. Each board within the NHS should put plans and arrangements in place to ensure that safe, effective and patient-focused care is being delivered and well supported. By understanding the infrastructure of clinical effectiveness, it is possible to appreciate the significant role that clinical audit plays in this process.

To support clinical effectiveness at each level, there is a range of quality improvement strategies and initiatives, such as:

• Guidelines and standards based on good evidence

• Quality improvement tools for monitoring and improving current practice

• Computerised information systems for facilitation of data storage and analysis

• Cost-effectiveness analysis/assessment tools

• Provision of learning and development opportunities across all levels of staff

The tools and support structures available for clinical effectiveness may be seen in the day-to-day provision of healthcare. The National Service Frameworks (NSFs) and the National Institute for Health and Clinical Excellence (NICE) are significant elements of clinical effectiveness; care pathways and local guidelines also contribute. Clinical audit forms one of the most essential tools for assessing and monitoring the standard of healthcare provision.

Role of clinical audit in clinical effectiveness

Clinical audit is a very effective tool for assessing the level of clinical effectiveness, and may achieve this by ensuring that all patients with a particular problem are treated with a procedure which fulfils a defined standard. It should be remembered that there may be other obstacles to efficient delivery of the service, such as insufficiently trained staff or lack of equipment. Clinical audit may also measure issues where standards have not been met and, with good data collection, identify the area hindering achievement. It can therefore be argued that clinical audit is paramount to achieving clinical effectiveness at all levels of clinical care delivered by the NHS and other healthcare institutions.

A good example of how national clinical audit has brought about clinical effectiveness is the Myocardial Infarction National Audit Project (MINAP). Cardiovascular disease is a major cause of mortality for the population in the UK and other parts of the world. The NSF for Coronary Heart Disease (CHD) was established in March 2000, and outlined the strategy for modernising CHD services over 10 years. It detailed 12 standards for improved prevention, diagnosis, treatment, rehabilitation and goals, and for securing fair access to high-quality services.

One of the main features within the standards was that patients who had an acute myocardial infarction fitting certain criteria were given thrombolysis within 60 minutes of calling for professional help. There had been well established research to show that thrombolysis helped to reduce mortality in such patients, and that the benefits of thrombolysis diminished with time after symptom onset. Earlier audits have shown that, in 2002, only 39% of eligible patients received thrombolytic therapy within 60 minutes (Boyle 2007). The results of these audits contributed to the remodelling of cardiac service delivery nationwide, with the introduction of priority response by ambulance services to patients with chest pain, and the appointment of cardiac nurse specialists to facilitate the procedure and treatment by paramedics. With the introduction of such strategies, numbers of patients treated within 60 minutes rose to more than 80%. This had in effect contributed to a substantial reduction in the 30-day mortality after myocardial infarction.

The audit also brought about improvements in the uptake of effective therapies on discharge after an acute myocardial infarction. Cardiac service delivery has been revolutionised by MINAP in the UK from all perspectives. Many other excellent examples of national audit put into practice (including the identification of deficits and targeting of resources) may be seen from the clinical care of patients with cancer, diabetes, renal failure and mental health problems, as set out in the respective NSFs.

Why do audit projects occasionally fail?

There are many occasions when clinical audits have been abandoned. This leads to a waste of resources and personnel. Even when completed, a project may not achieve what was set out initially. There are many pitfalls worthy of discussion.

Poor preparation

Most mistakes are made at this stage. The selection of an audit topic is often seen as an easy task; however the end result may not yield the quality of results to impact on clinical effectiveness. When an audit topic does not affirm an evidence-based standard or a well recognised guideline, there is a risk that the definition of 'good practice' will be debated. Poorly defined standards may occasionally hinder the progress of an audit project.

Even a carefully selected audit topic may not be relevant in all situations. Certain standards apply specifically to particular populations and may not be applied in all contexts. For example, a certain imaging technique may be an excellent tool for diagnosis and therefore may be advocated as the first-line investigation; however some smaller hospitals in rural areas may not have the resources or expertise to provide such a service to all patients.

Good support for the planning and execution of an audit project is not always obtained. Many local NHS organisations have an audit department that is able to facilitate data acquisition and analysis, and provide advice with regard to process; this facility is often underused. In addition, junior doctors normally need supervision from clinicians more experienced at clinical audit. If help from clinicians and the Clinical Audit Department is not sought initially, the audit project may progress inefficiently having been poorly planned.

Poor execution

Clinical audit may be conducted either prospectively or retrospectively. On occasions, the investigator may not begin to understand the way in which the audit project should be conducted. Some projects need to be completed prospectively, as certain critical information may not have been recorded earlier.

It is essential when collecting data to think about the 'what', 'where' and 'who'. Some data may not be easy to obtain. This may be a consequence of complex accessibility or the need for consent from the patient. The resulting lengthy process may discourage the investigator after commencement. The location of the information also needs to be well considered. If the individuals who are delegated to collect the data are not able to differentiate between appropriate, correct and unimportant material, there will be a risk of acquiring erroneous or insufficient data.

Failure to implement change and re-audit

On occasions, even though deficiencies in the system may be identified on presentation, there is failure to implement the changes after the audit. The implementation of change can be rather difficult if there is a lot of resistance from different groups of people involved in the delivery of care. Lack of implementation, irrespective of the preceding good work, may therefore equate to a failed audit.

After implementation, re-audit is essential in order to ensure that improvement is seen and to complete the initial audit cycle. One should never assume that improvement will occur; some of the implementations may not have any impact at all, or may create new problems that prevent the standards being met.

Examples of good practice for clinical audit

Some general pointers, which are reinforced throughout this book and which play a prominent role in the production of a successful clinical audit project, include:

- Recognition of clinical audit as a vital component of clinical practice; this may include the provision of protected time for clinicians

- Support from a larger body, for example strategic health authority, Care Quality Commission (CQC)

- Partnership with skilled professionals, clinical and non-clinical, outside the immediate clinical field (this should include nursing staff, therapists and managers); partnership and good liaisons with patients; partnership across the primary/secondary care interface

- High-level evidence for guidelines

- Availability of high quality information technology and good quality patient records

Good examples of clinical audit

Countless clinical audits are conducted every day throughout the country, though they greatly vary in quality. Below are examples of successful audits.

In an acute environment such as the admission ward in a hospital, clinical audit can make a rapid difference to the standard of treatment. Patients frequently present with acute shortness of breath as the primary complaint. One of the main differential diagnoses to be considered may include pulmonary embolism, where immediate treatment could be critical. As it is well established that low-molecular-weight heparin is the best evidence-based treatment for reducing mortality from pulmonary embolism, a gold standard could be the immediate treatment of a suspected case with low-molecular-weight heparin unless contraindicated. Compliance with this standard may be measured using clinical audit. Data collection is easily obtained, prospectively or retrospectively, by looking at drug prescriptions and clinical notes. If a deficiency in treatment of patients with suspected pulmonary embolism exists, problems will surface and changes may be implemented to improve the system. This should be followed with re-audit. This is a good example of a local audit with evidence-based practice, and a standard that is achievable and effective.

At the national level, a wide range of audits is conducted, mainly through government initiatives or healthcare professionals' organisations, such as The Royal Colleges, NSFs, healthcare institutions and patients' associations. As a rule these national clinical audits are very well organised in order to improve patient care throughout the whole country. An excellent example is the National Sentinel Stroke Audit, which is driven by The Royal College of Physicians and looks at the care for stroke patients throughout the whole of England, Wales and Northern Ireland. This audit was started in 1998 and has taken place every 2 years. It looks at many aspects of management in stroke patients from investigations and acute care to rehabilitation, including the location of management (the gold standard being that the management of strokes confers better mortality when located in a specialised stroke unit). This audit has set national guidelines for every hospital to follow; improvement has been seen on the occasion of each re-audit, and targets have gradually become more stringent. For example, in 2002, only 72% of hospitals had an acute stroke unit, but this improved with changes to 94% in 2006 (Clinical Effectiveness and Evaluation Unit 2006).

Successful audit: who will benefit?

A successful audit will benefit all stakeholders

Patients

Patients are the main beneficiaries of clinical audit because the latter is mainly performed in healthcare services to monitor and improve the standards of healthcare delivery. This ensures that patients are always managed according to agreed guidelines, which are mostly evidence based. The constant review of guidelines should lead to improvement in many facets of care, ranging from mortality and satisfaction to administration.

Healthcare professionals

Doctors and other healthcare professionals will all benefit from a successful project, often simply by acquiring experience and exposure to clinical audit. There is a great opportunity for self-improvement. New and useful skills may be learned, such as computing, information technology, statistical knowledge, project design, organisational skills, team working, leadership and management. A successful clinical audit can develop a team of well rounded healthcare professionals.

Healthcare management personnel

As clinical effectiveness implies the usage of appropriate evidence-based practice in the most cost-effective way to provide the best outcome, so, in many circumstances, successful clinical audit can contribute to good cost-effective clinical care delivery. Cost-effectiveness can also be achieved when a successful clinical audit rectifies a poor practice method and increases efficiency to attain the recommended standards.

Public

A good quality clinical audit serves as excellent feedback to the public on the status of healthcare service delivery. Hard facts and figures may facilitate comparison between individuals and institutions and this may in turn impact on patient behaviour, as seen with the choose-and-book system.

Informative clinical audits may help to identify both the successes and failures of a system. The identification of 'failures' may generate increased public awareness, thereby creating a driver for change.

National bodies and national clinical audits

In 2006, the Chief Medical Officer produced a report *Good Doctors, Safer Patients*. In this report, he called for the reinvigoration of clinical audit to maximise its potential in providing an excellent assessment tool to support clinical effectiveness in patient care. The 2007 White Paper, 'Trust, Assurance and Safety', also concurred with this aspiration. This led to the conception of some national bodies charged with the development of clinical audit.

National Clinical Audit Advisory Group (NCAAG)

After the recommendations from the Chief Medical Officer's report, the National Clinical Audit Advisory Group (NCAAG) was established to drive the reinvigoration programme and provide a national focus for discussion and advice on matters relating to clinical audit. This launch marked the effort that the Department of

Health put into promoting national audits at the centre of the NHS. Today, NCAAG has huge responsibilities to expand any existing programme of national audits and integrate it into local audits of individual trusts by supporting the NHS workers. This group seeks to improve connections between central and local matters, as well as intercalating research and development, revalidation and information technology developments.

The NCAAG will also be the steering group for the expanded National Clinical Audit and Patients' Outcomes Programme (NCAPOP). The functions of NCAAG may be summarised as follows:

- To reinvigorate clinical audit, both nationally and locally, yielding new publicly available information to support improvements to clinical practice and service delivery.

- To be the steering group for the NCAPOP, providing advice and guidance on the overall programme of work, and in particular to consider proposals for new audits or for discontinuation of existing audits.

- To advise on some additional issues as requested by the Department of Health:

  1. To recommend how the Connecting for Health programme can best support national and local audit

  2. To advise on the interface of clinical audit with revalidation

  3. To advise on the integration of local audits with NHS litigation authority

National Clinical Audit and Patient Outcome Programme (NCAPOP)

The NCAPOP was in the past hosted by the Healthcare Commission.

The current new host is a consortium made up of the Academy of Medical Royal Colleges, The Royal College of Nursing and the Healthcare Quality Improvement Partnership (HQIP). This consortium has the responsibility of expanding the current programme, which includes commissioning national audits across a range of specialties; the programme as a whole included over 20 active audits, and the expanded programme includes the following:

- Commissioning national audits: prioritising topics on the basis of advice from the NCAAG. The audit programme will be expanded to incorporate two national audits that currently sit outside the programme (the National Joint Registry and the Paediatric Intensive Care audit), and it is expected that further new audits will be developed.

- Stakeholder engagement: consultation with stakeholders, including clinicians, professional organisations, users of audit and others, will be an essential part of reinvigorating audit and building consensus on how to develop audit in the future. This will be the key to forging a productive national clinical audit programme, and linking effectively with local audit. The NCAPOP will establish a wide and inclusive stakeholder forum as one means of enabling discussion and debate.

- Support for clinical audit: the NCAPOP will have new responsibilities to develop materials and resources to support practitioners carrying out both local and national audits. These might include training materials and guidance, and a library of validated audits that practitioners can download for use locally.

Healthcare Quality Improvement Partnership (HQIP)

This body is led by a consortium of the Academy of Medical Royal Colleges, Royal College of Nursing and National Voices (formerly the Long-term Conditions Alliance), and is designed to promote better health services by supporting those responsible for quality improvement work.

It was established in April 2008 to promote quality in healthcare, and in particular to increase the impact that clinical audit has on healthcare quality in England and Wales. It aims to support local staff, promotes active dissemination of information and implements quality improvement initiatives. There is a remit in England and Wales to commission national clinical audits (and also to promote local clinical audit in England). There is currently no remit in Scotland or Northern Ireland, although those who are working in clinical audit in these areas, or who are working in local clinical audit in Wales, may download any content from the HQIP site. The agency hosts the contract to manage and develop the National Clinical Audit and Patient Outcomes Programme (NCAPOP).

The Royal Colleges

The Royal College of Physicians have discussed the role of clinical audit within clinical practice and have stressed the following points.

- Improving the quality of care: the results of audits should be reviewed within departments and used to inform efforts at service development.

- Audit as part of routine practice: the increasing development of information technology within the NHS should provide the opportunity for routine clinical data gathering to feed into clinical audit processes.

- Getting the patient's perspective: clinical audit should develop to ensure that the patient's perspective is included in assessing the quality of service provided.

- Training: clinical audit should provide an opportunity to learn the principles of literature searching and critical appraisal as well as issues of data collection and change management.

- Revalidation: the government White Paper *Trust Assurance and Safety* (Department of Health, 2007) proposes that audit should play an important part in revalidation. It is important that clinicians participate in audit and demonstrate that they have reflected on its outcomes.

Interestingly, two of these five points relate to training and ongoing assessment of doctors, showing the value that The Royal Colleges place on the practice of audit not only to improve quality and safety in healthcare but also to train and assess competencies among doctors.

As a result of their commitment to clinical audit the Royal College of Physicians have coordinated several collaborative audits though their Clinical Effectiveness and Evaluation Unit (CEEU). The aim of the CEEU is to ensure that best practice and evidence-based approaches to care are widely disseminated and used for the benefit of patients. It achieves this by producing national clinical guidelines, designing national comparative clinical audit tools to evaluate standards of organisation and delivery of clinical care, and coordinating national comparative clinical audit projects. As a group they have completed several audit projects, including one on lung cancer, a national sentinel audit of stroke, evidence-based prescribing for older people, multiple sclerosis 360° audit and the myocardial infarction national audit project. Their ongoing projects include chronic obstructive pulmonary disease (COPD), continence, and falls and bone health. In addition they have developed guidelines for clinical practice from the audit work that they have undertaken such as the national clinical guideline for stroke.

The Royal College of Surgeons have been equally active in advocating the practice of clinical audit. They have developed methodologies for clinical audit in dentistry and guidelines for clinical audit in surgical practice.

National clinical audits

These projects should meet all the following criteria:

- National coverage (in England) should be either achieved or intended

- The main focus should be on the quality of clinical practice

- Clinical practice should be evaluated against criteria/guidelines and/or outcome data

- The audit cycle should be applied, and/or clinical/patient outcome data should be monitored in an ongoing way

- Projects should be conducted prospectively (for example retrospective reviews of adverse outcomes such as confidential enquiries are not included)

- Projects should include patients and their governance; data is taken from patients themselves

National clinical audit is designed to improve patient outcomes across a wide range of medical, surgical and mental health conditions. Its purpose is to engage all healthcare professionals across England and Wales in systematic evaluation of their clinical practice against standards, and to support and encourage improvement in the quality of treatment and care.

Most national clinical audits have been developed because they are in a highly important area of medicine and one where it is felt that national results are essential to improve practice and standards. In all cases they form part of a broader approach to improve quality, and fit into the information strategy of the condition involved. This is particularly relevant in areas such as cancer or diabetes, which have national information strategies.

Such audits are backed by the relevant Royal College and the national clinical director concerned; they usually have the support and involvement of the relevant national voluntary organisation that represents patient interests.

In summary, national clinical audit is established through the Department of Health's initiative to ensure that delivery of care in the NHS achieves the highest standards. This should be achieved by setting out a national programme, run by a consortium consisting of the general public, patients and healthcare professionals.

Key points

- Clinical effectiveness is the framework for using the most cost-effective evidence-based practice in healthcare service delivery to obtain the maximum outcome benefit

- Clinical audit is the best tool for assessing clinical effectiveness, and therefore plays a pivotal role in the current modern NHS climate

- Clinical audit can fail when there is poor preparation, poor execution and failure to implement changes and re-audit

- Some factors for successful clinical audit include:

  1. Recognition of clinical audit as a vital component of clinical practice

  2. Support from a larger body

  3. Partnership with skilled professionals outside the immediate clinical field

  4. Partnership and good liaisons with patients

  5. Partnership across the primary/secondary care interface

  6. High level evidence for guidelines

7. Availability of high quality information technology and good quality patient records

- Successful clinical audits benefit everyone, most importantly patients, healthcare professionals, healthcare management personnel and the public in general

- In response to the Chief Medical Officer's report *Good Doctors, Safer Patients* in 2006, many national bodies, charged with the development of clinical audit, emerged

- National clinical audits are established to ensure that quality of clinical care is achieved and standardised throughout the whole country

References

Academy of Medical Royal Colleges (2007). *The Foundation Programme: Curriculum,* London.

Boyle R. (2007). *Coronary Heart Disease Ten Years On – Improving Heart Care Report*, Department of Health, London.

Clinical Effectiveness and Evaluation Unit (2006). *National Sentinel Stroke Audit*. Royal College of Physicians.

Department of Health (2007). The White Paper *Trust, Assurance and Safety – The Regulation of Health Professionals in the 21st Century*, The Stationery Office, London.

NHS Executive (1996). *Promoting Clinical Effectiveness – A framework for action in and through the NHS*, Department of Health, London.

The Chief Medical Officer (2006). *Good Doctors, Safer Patients*. Department of Health, London.

Chapter 3 The sources of support for clinical audit within and outside the trust

Embarking on a clinical audit project may be daunting even for the experienced auditor. It is therefore important to plan carefully and identify support. There are many people who may be able to advise and support, and this is discussed below. Before embarking on an audit, it is vital that plans are discussed with the local audit department (if available). Many clinical audit departments formally register all audit projects, in order to maintain control of the quality and numbers of ongoing projects, maintain awareness of all outcomes and prevent duplication of work.

Resources

It is important to treat the start of an audit project with respect; this will involve careful thought with regard to resources and planning.

A firm grasp of information technology is very important. It would be useful (some would say vital) to have access to a computer at home and at work. Programs should be compatible to allow daily updating of spreadsheets and data preservation. Problems of confidentiality and data loss may be overcome with the use of an encrypted removable storage device. Multiple copies of pro formas and questionnaires should be stored; access to suitable copying and/ or printing facilities is therefore paramount.

When researching possible projects for audit, internet searches (for example PubMed or Cochrane databases) may be essential, as is access to medical journals, particularly when analysing the results.

Increasingly journals are becoming available online and many can be accessed through hospital websites. Local medical libraries are vital when required journals are only available in print.

General stationery and equipment to undertake the audit is essential.

Most clinical audit projects do not need funding, however occasionally specific equipment or computer programs may be required, which may prove expensive. When presenting results, travelling to conferences and printing posters can also incur costs.

Funding implications for the trust

It should be recognised that a successful clinical audit project and ensuing implementation may either decrease trust/hospital costs (through improved efficiency) or increase costs (through providing extra resources for improved quality). The scenario of future increased expenditure should be recognised as early as possible, as the trust board may wish to consider the implications and identify the pressures for achieving and not achieving the relevant standard. In general, clinical audits which have the potential of improving quality should be financially supported, as the benefits to the trust are wide and varied (including improved patient satisfaction, commissioning satisfaction and the achievement of 'target' standards.)

Funding for projects

When assessing the need for funding for the project, the benefits to the trust (dealt with in the preceding paragraph) should be made clear to the individuals or board responsible for funding. This is particularly relevant for cases where future increased efficiency may lead to decreased expenditure. It is possible that as the drive for quality accelerates, trust boards may actually lead discussions for cost-inducing projects.

There may be multiple sources of funding in most trusts, though they can be difficult to navigate. A good starting point is the discussion of funding issues with your potential audit team (senior *and* junior colleagues) and the clinical audit department. The latter will certainly either have some direct funding (however small) or the knowledge and expertise to re-direct funding applications.

There may be additional external sources of funding available from the national bodies specialising in clinical audit mentioned in Chapter 2. In addition the Royal Colleges, Royal Society of Medicine and other learned societies occasionally have funds; this is usually for research although not exclusively so. Websites should be checked carefully, and one should be vigilant of advertisements in medical journals or website notice boards. All funding applications need to be made in good time; the process is often lengthy.

Sources of support

Clinical support

By working as part of a firm, and often as part of a much larger multidisciplinary team including nursing staff, therapists and pharmacists, doctors have on tap a great array of valuable sources of information and advice when planning an audit.

The consultant will have a significant interest in the standard and quality of healthcare provided by the firm for patients who may be under his or her care. An awareness of new guidelines introduced to the hospital, or alternatively an observation of a problem, may therefore lead to frequent ideas for 'top-down' projects. If 'ready-made' projects are not forthcoming, junior doctors should have shown initiative by identifying triggers for potential audits. Indeed, when requesting guidance from a senior colleague with regard to audit topic selection, individuals should be prepared to have the question thrown back at them: 'You have been on the firm now for 3 weeks, tell me something we could do better … tell me about an area you would like to audit … tell me about an area we should audit?' A fundamental understanding of the clinical audit process should lead to the identification of relatively simple projects.

Once a project is under way, the status and ongoing issues should always be discussed by way of progress updates with the whole clinical audit team and other stakeholders (for example key clinicians and other multidisciplinary members). Progress meetings may in turn lead to useful suggestions for improvements, help with choosing venues for presentation (and indeed help with publication).

It is worth remembering that discussions and feedback from more junior team members may be as useful as those from senior colleagues. Often, simple housekeeping and practical issues may be identified, leading to the saving of invaluable time.

Undertaking an audit in groups of at least three splits the workload and provides different perspectives, though clearly one-man projects on occasions have succeeded and will continue to thrive. It is important to ensure that the lead auditor has the impetus to complete the project, and that all the fellow auditors have an assigned role.

Non-clinical support

One of the issues that people find most challenging is data analysis. After careful collection of a huge amount of data many projects go no further, usually as a consequence of a lack of confidence with regard to statistical analysis. The project is therefore left unanalysed and not presented. Alternatively data may be partially analysed by looking solely at numerical trends rather than at statistics.

If a complete statistical analysis is not undertaken, it is often impossible to detect whether the trends are truly significant. It also makes it difficult to compare audit results with published data. Hence it is beneficial to discuss issues with experts in the local statistics department. They may be in a position to provide simple advice, or even manual help with the data analysis. Many hospitals are attached to medical schools and universities, which have research centres and statistics departments.

Secretaries and ward clerks are on numerous occasions invaluable to audit projects. They are intimately familiar with the processes of ordering and tracking down notes, which differs from institution to institution. Occasionally data is more readily retrieved from electronic patient records; the information technology department may be helpful if there are particular issues.

Research specialist nurses are generally involved with the organisation of research and clinical trials and are experienced in data collection, analysis and applications to ethics committees.

Literature search skills should be developed by becoming familiar with commonly used databases; in times of difficulty, the hospital librarian will prove a valuable resource.

Local clinical audit department

The roles of the clinical audit department are multiple. The primary responsibility is to advise and provide a strategic overview of clinical audit activity within the Trust. Often, the department will be responsible not only for clinical audit, but also the larger remit of clinical effectiveness. This may include the overseeing of necessary processes in order to ensure that the highest standards of clinical care are achieved, monitored and maintained. In order to do this effectively the department requires systems to register audits, collect statistical information about audits and publish regular reports. These reports may be annual or more frequent, and aimed at the trust or any third party.

A rolling programme of audits should be undertaken to provide assurance that the trust is providing a high quality service. This information should be stored in a database that is available to all staff. The audit department may also follow up projects to ensure that changes have been implemented and re-audits have been undertaken or planned. It is also able to promote pieces of work to ensure that the lessons learned are shared among other departments where the data may be relevant. All of this strengthens the process of audit and perpetuates the drive towards the improvement of patient care.

Key components of the clinical audit process should be tracked by the department, in order to ensure quality outcomes and also to demonstrate key clinical audit process standards to any third party. This should also allow the capture of any shortfall in training, awareness or support.

The Chair of the department is usually a nominated consultant who takes overall clinical responsibility for the functions of the committee. This person is the key conduit between clinicians and executives, by providing assurance to the trust that high quality effective care is being achieved through clinical audit.

The clinical audit manager provides operational support to the department by maintaining and monitoring the processes for clinical audit. Training staff, identifying audit requirements, initiating audit, providing support to clinical auditors and monitoring implementation of guidelines are all part of this role. He or she should report on audit activity and national guideline implementation, and routinely present the latter at each departmental meeting. Therefore all audit activity should be captured on the trust system, which in turn should facilitate all projects to be completed and recommendations made in a timely manner. This information may be used as evidence to the Care Quality Commission and other bodies to demonstrate the meeting of national standards.

The clinical audit department should also incorporate a manager from each directorate who is responsible for audit. These individuals should receive regular reports regarding audit activity at a directorate level, and provide links and support between the clinical areas, the directorate and clinical audit department. There should also be directorate and specialty clinical leads for audit.

Typical clinical audit committee meetings, therefore, are attended by the Chair, the clinical audit manager, directorate managers and clinical audit leads.

Clinical audit departments may also provide some general assistance:

- When individuals present themselves to clinical audit departments without a proposed topic, the department may be in a position to point them in the direction of ongoing audits, or towards audit leads

- They may be a good source of ideas for novel audits

- Most audit departments will help to find standards or guidelines that are relevant to a registered audit

- They may help to develop patient questionnaires and pro formas, be in a position to request notes or occasionally help with data analysis and presentations

- After presentation of the data, they will also facilitate an action plan for implementation of changes and set a timescale for a schedule for re-audit (see Addendum A below.)

The multi-faceted support structure described here may be summarised in an audit handbook, either in the form of hard copies, or available electronically.

Registering the audit project with the local audit department

All audits should be registered with the audit department. As mentioned at the beginning of this chapter, registration is vital to enable audit departments to take control of all audit projects and prevent duplication of work. It is unfortunate that only a minority are in fact registered; this may be explained by a lack of awareness of the process or time pressures. In some trusts it is now mandatory to register audits.

Some audit departments provide a registration pack that includes all the necessary information to register the project, together with some general advice. An example of a clinical audit registration form is available in Addendum B below.

Research and development office

It is not a common requirement to contact the research and development office while completing an audit project. However, audits may occasionally lead to novel research, so it is important that its role and position within the organisation is understood.

The research and development department supports high-quality research and development within the trust. It aims to support researchers and facilitate links between departments, universities, industries, ethics committees and local research networks. The office processes research applications for trust approval and provides advice to researchers on matters relating to research governance. It monitors all research activities within the trust and provides advice on funding opportunities and grant applications. Importantly it oversees the implementation of national policies, which are designed to improve the quality of research by protecting patients and staff, ensuring scientific quality and maximising the impact of research. Annual reports are produced for the Department of Health and collaborations with research councils, universities, research networks and commercial companies are formed. The office identifies research and development training needs of all trust staff and develops training programmes to meet this need. It ensures that all research conducted within the trust is accounted for and is on the research and development register. It also works with the trust directorates to advocate embedding research and research findings into clinical practice.

The registration of research projects involving trust patients is usually a relatively lengthy process requiring submission of a range of documents including an ethics application form, consent, copy of the study protocol, evidence of funding and indemnity.

The organisation of clinical audit in locations without audit departments

Hospitals increasingly have greater autonomy over how they organise themselves and supply services. As a result some trusts have changed the way that they govern audit, and now occasionally fragment audit projects into relevant directorates or divisions; this may occur with or without the facility of a central database of all registered projects. When clinical audit is fragmented in this way, receiving advice and support may be challenging. It is particularly relevant in these cases to draw on other clinical and non-clinical sources of support, as highlighted elsewhere. Hospital trusts, no matter how they organise audit, have a way of registering audit projects and it is important that this is still undertaken. If there is no audit department, sources of help may include the clinical governance department or the audit officer in your own department or directorate.

External sources of support

There are sources of support outside the trust that may be able to deal with queries and provide support for the project.

NICE

The National Institute for Health and Clinical Excellence (NICE) have produced a high quality piece of work entitled *Principles for Best Practice in Clinical Audit* (2002.) These guidelines were developed to help NHS trusts and individuals determine whether practice is in accordance with NICE guidance.

The Clinical Audit Support Centre

The Clinical Audit Support Centre (CASC) was set up in 2006. As the organisers of the group had previously been managers of audit in a primary care group, they had a significant amount of experience of clinical audit and quality assurance across defined sectors of the NHS.

The main aim of the centre is to provide quality assured support and training to healthcare professionals across a range of quality improvement fields. It endeavours to facilitate and support audits that improve patient care and enhance service delivery. Trusts are assisted with strategic support; this includes the setting up of major new initiatives such as involvement of patients in clinical audit. Individuals who are struggling with an audit project may be assisted. It is important to remember that CASC is a private company which charges for the support provided. Payment of a fee will lead to the allocation of a designated adviser who will work exclusively with you throughout the whole project, including aftercare and follow up. Although this service may seem too expensive for standard clinical audit projects, it may be invaluable for primary care and hospital trusts for the purposes of reorganising clinical audit and assisting with large-scale projects.

Key points

- Be aware of resources and plan properly
- A successful clinical audit project and ensuing implementation may either decrease trust/hospital costs (through improved efficiency) or increase costs (through providing extra resources for improved quality)
- There may be multiple sources of funding in most trusts, though they can be difficult to navigate. A good starting

point is the discussion of funding issues with your potential audit team and the clinical audit department. The latter will certainly either have some direct funding or the knowledge and expertise to redirect funding applications.

- Clinical support: primarily from clinical audit team
- Non clinical support
  - Local clinical audit department
  - Research and development office advice may be relevant
  - External sources for support

Further reading

National Institute for Health and Clinical Excellence (2002). *Principles for Best Practice in Clinical Audit*, Radcliffe Medical Press Ltd, Oxford.

Addendum A
Clinical audit project action plan

Title of clinical audit project:

....

Directorate: ....

Date: ....

Recommended change in practice	Plan	Date to be completed by.	Completed Yes/ No
1.			
2.			
3.			
4.			
5.			
6.			

Addendum B
Clinical audit registration form

Complete and return to the Clinical Audit Manager. You will receive an authorisation number when the project has been registered. **You should not proceed with your project until this is completed and you will not be able to request notes without this.**

Title and short summary of project

Reason for project

Objective of audit

Keywords: please provide keywords relating to your audit to assist those searching on the intranet. (For example, "Audit of the management of asthma patients in A&E against national guidelines" might be found by searching under the keyword "asthma" or "A&E". If this is a Patient and Public Involvement Project "PPI" should be a keyword.)

Person(s) carrying out the project
Name(s)

Position(s)

Specialty/department

Telephone

E-mail

Division:

☐   Children, Women and Sexual Health

☐   Diagnostics, Surgery and Outpatients

☐   General and Emergency Medicine

☐   Trust wide

Project Supervisor (this should be the supervising individual who carries senior responsibility for the project)

Name

Position

Telephone

E-mail

Audit governance risk

☐   Risk of anonymity preservation

☐   Patient consent required

Further details of any governance implications

```
```

Triggers which prompted this clinical audit project

- ☐ Perception: e.g. there is local concern or there may be wide variation in practice
- ☐ Adverse event
- ☐ Patient Outcome Monitoring: complaints, experiences and perceived outcome.
- ☐ National Guideline (e.g. NICE, NSF, Royal College)
- ☐ National Diktat – A mandatory audit from a national authoritative body
- ☐ Local guideline, process or committee
- ☐ Local diktat – The Trust attaches importance to a national/local guideline and makes an audit mandatory.
- ☐ Re-audit of previous audit
- ☐ Other, please state:

```
```

Impact

- ☐ Personal practice
- ☐ Local practice
- ☐ Regional/national practice
- ☐ Auditing high risk intervention
- ☐ Auditing high volume intervention
- ☐ Auditing high cost intervention

Title of source of standard or guideline

```
```

Priority of project

- ☐ National
- ☐ Regional
- ☐ Departmental consensus
- ☐ Trust consensus

Involvement (including advice or funding) from national bodies
- ☐ Royal Colleges
- ☐ HQIP
- ☐ NCAPOP
- ☐ NCAAG
- ☐ SHA
- ☐ CQC
- ☐ Clinical Audit Support Centre

Is any other support required? If so please state:

```



```

What methods will be used (e.g. for data collection)?

```




```

Will access be required to medical records for notes retrieval?

```


```

Start date of project

```

```

Target completion date

```

```

Signatures

Signature of lead auditor

Date:

Signature of Project Supervisor (mandatory)

Date:

Signature of Assistant General Manager – Quality and Risk (mandatory)

Date:

Office use only

Date registered:

Chapter 4   Triggers for clinical audits

We have seen that clinical audits may be conducted in many facets of healthcare. Projects driven from a clinical perspective may include waiting times, administrative documentation and clinical standards for treatment; operational projects may encompass cost-effectiveness and targets.

It is vital that the concept of 'triggers' is grasped. The categorisation of the prompt at the outset of a project will facilitate:

- The focussing of the mind for all clinical auditors

- A method for retrospectively analysing 'all reasons for' performing clinical audit

- A demonstration to third parties that the path to clinical effectiveness and quality is mapped out. The categorisation of all triggers should therefore confirm that the clinical audit projects have been driven by a need rather than a tick box process.

This chapter will explore various triggers, as briefly outlined here:

- Perception: there may be a perceived notion that an activity needs to be audited (either because it is performed badly or well)

- Adverse event: an incident or series of incidences may highlight a deficiency in clinical practice

- National Guideline: most clinicians would agree that it is good practice to assess national standards within a rolling programme.

These may originate from a learned society or any other body, and become apparent at a convention, seminar, journals or by other correspondence. Increasingly, trusts are pro-actively seeking to capture high profile national guidelines (for example NICE guidelines) and auditing against them if they are relevant to practice

- National diktat: a mandatory audit may be required from a national authoritative body (for example, NPSA, Department of Health, Care Quality Commission)

- Local guideline, process or committee: it is good practice to audit against local standards within a rolling programme. Many of these standards may also be national guidelines. Many local processes and committees are vital for standards, and may provide ammunition for clinical audit

- Local diktat: The trust attaches sufficient importance to a national or local guideline, and makes the audit against this standard mandatory.

Indeed most forums, including academic meetings and local committees (for example those dealing with risk, complaints, patient satisfaction, hygiene, security, pharmacy and nutrition) should include an agenda item: 'Should this be audited?'

Figure 4.1, 4.2 and 4.3 graphically display the pathways related to some of the aforementioned triggers. These should be referred to in conjunction with the rest of this chapter.

Perception as a trigger to audit

Many aspects of day-to-day practice may impact on your perception of quality. Some important examples are discussed here.

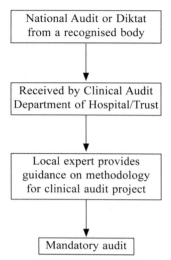

Figure 4.1   **National audit or diktat as trigger**

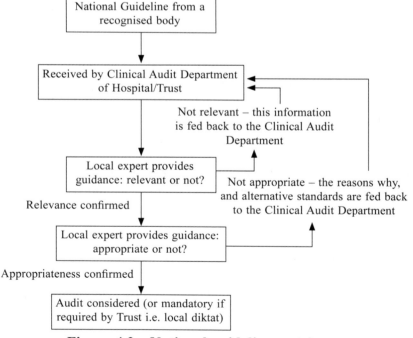

Figure 4.2   **National guideline as trigger**

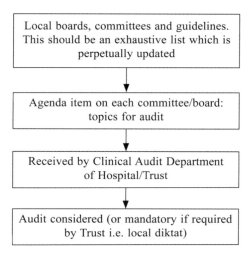

Figure 4.3   Local boards, committees and guidelines as triggers

Recurring clinical problems

This is a common issue. When a problem is spotted, a clinical audit may be designed with specific standards in place.

A common example is hospital inpatient falls, which have huge implications, contributing as they do to a delay in recovery, clinical complications and an increase in costs. This is a clinical problem that has caught the attention of the public and also healthcare professionals. Therefore, the NPSA has conducted a data set compilation to look at this problem. The Executive Summary, *Slips, Trips and Falls in Hospital* (2007) estimated that patients falling in hospitals cost the NHS around £15 million every year. This is evident when we can see that the National Reporting and Learning System (NRSL) reported over 200,000 falls between September 2005 and August 2006, resulting in hip fractures, broken bones and even death. Recommendations have since been put forward to reduce such incidents from a multidisciplinary point of view.

From a local perspective, a clinical audit can be developed if hospital inpatient falls are known to be a major problem. This may be identified for example by the night duty team. The identification of the specific clinical problem and the incorporation of local protocols and NPSA recommendations as standards may lead to a feasible clinical audit to enable a change in practice. The standards and changes may range from ensuring sufficient staff and providing a suitable environment for older, confused patients.

Feedback

On occasions, healthcare professionals underestimate the importance of feedback, particularly from patients and relatives (as well as from healthcare staff). Feedback is received by most doctors, almost on a daily basis. Persistent and similar feedback in a particular area may alert the doctor that something is amiss, and could relate to a simple oversight that has failed to be identified by healthcare professionals.

A common example can be related to preoperative assessment and consent for an operation. Preoperative assessment is standard practice in healthcare, to improve safety and efficiency. Patients (perhaps with the help of their families) need to have sufficient information about the operative risks and benefits, together with information about the anaesthesia, before making a decision about an operation. It is not unusual for patients and their family members to feed back that the information is insufficient and often too late (often immediately preceding the seeking of consent). Feedback such as this should heighten awareness and lead to the identification of standards. This in turn may prompt the formation of a new protocol to ensure the provision of timely and comprehensive information, and the value of consent. This may then be audited.

Direct observation of care

An error or issue may be directly observed. This has provided the catalyst for many national clinical audit projects. The measurement of 'vital observations' may be a relevant example.

Patients' vital signs of blood pressure, heart rate, respiratory rate and oxygen saturation are important physiological measurements and are measured at varying frequencies for most patients in hospital. They often serve as early warning signs of deterioration of a patient's condition before they manifest clinically. However, one frequently witnesses a lack of consistency in documenting these parameters, even in acutely ill patients.

The Modified Early Warning Score (MEWS) is a tool for bedside evaluation based on these physiological parameters, with a numerical score attached to the degree of deviation of each physiological response from the norm. It is often considered good practice that a certain score triggers an intervention and escalation of clinical care when appropriate.

It is therefore reasonable to perform a clinical audit project to assess whether all acutely unwell patients have consistent vital sign monitoring, documentation of an appropriate MEWS score is made, and appropriate action is taken.

Adverse event (and near miss)

An adverse event was defined in the white paper *Organisation with a Memory* (NHS Report 2000) as:

'An event or omission arising during clinical care and causing physical and psychological injury to a patient'.

Near misses, on the other hand, were defined in the same paper as:

'A situation in which an event or omission or a sequence of events or omissions arising during clinical care fails to develop further, whether or not as the result of compensating actions, thus preventing injury to the patient'.

In some trusts, near misses are divided into two types:

1. True near misses: harm is prevented as a result of the error being identified and ensuring preventative action.

2. Harm does not occur, simply due to chance (rather than intervention.)

All acute trusts now have mandatory reporting systems enabling all individuals including medical staff to be alerted to adverse events or near misses. As a general rule, adverse events require mandatory reporting, as serious harm may result in illness, dissatisfaction, fines, negative publicity or legal action against the healthcare organisation. Near misses, however, often surface only through voluntary reporting. It is important to recognise that it is through such reporting systems that deficiencies in healthcare service may be identified and improved.

Therefore it is also important to understand the various methods of reporting adverse events. The patient safety literature contains a number of examples:

- Anonymous mail

- Confidential mail

- Open-ended narratives

- Electronic input (may include pre-coded drop-down menus).

There is little evidence to indicate which methods improve reporting rates.

By understanding the operational pathways undertaken during the adverse incident pathway, the relevance of clinical audit triggers may be recognised. After review of the report by the risk department, one may with the aid of assisted reports from colleagues within the trust, identify issues and errors. A conclusion is drafted, and a new local protocol may also be created. This provides the standard against which an audit project may be commenced.

It is probable that near misses lead to less formal investigations; this would depend on the methods of presentation and collation of near miss reports. On occasions the rigid compliance with good protocols and guidelines may nevertheless lead to true near misses, as the absence of the protocol may have in other circumstances led to actual harm. A good case in point is that of the error-rich field of drug prescriptions, where vigilance processes are in place with constant regulations and updates. Drug prescription errors for example, may be spotted by the dispenser, and a feedback mechanism may be in place to clarify the prescription. A clinical audit project may test the robustness of such a process.

National diktat

A mandatory audit may be required by a national authoritative body (for example the Care Quality Commission, National Patient Safety Agency, NHS Litigation Authority). The topic in question, which inevitably relates to national standards, is clearly seen as vital, and is cascaded to all trusts. The responsible trust manager is charged with the responsibility for re-cascading the topic to the relevant specialist (by way of the audit lead in the directorate or department). A response, including the projected date for commencing and completing the audit project, is fed back to the clinical audit department, who in turn informs the responsible external body.

National guideline

Most clinicians would agree that it is good practice to assess national standards within a rolling programme. These may originate from a learned society or any other body, and become apparent in a convention, seminar, journal or by other correspondence.

As these high profile guidelines will impact greatly on clinical care, and because it is likely that more and more national guidelines will become 'national diktats' (see above), trusts are beginning to seek proactively to capture high profile national guidelines (for example NICE guidelines) in order to consider them for clinical audit projects. Some indeed are converted into 'local diktats' (see below). The clinical audit department may cascade the considered guideline to a relevant specialist (by way of the audit lead in the directorate or department) who is then asked to comment on whether the guideline is relevant to practice. If it is relevant, comments are provided on the degree of appropriateness. If wholly appropriate, it may be prudent to adopt the guideline (if not already adopted) and audit against it. If partially or wholly not appropriate, comments may indicate why this should be, and steps should be taken to identify which guideline is currently used in preference to the considered guideline. It would be good practice to adopt the preferred guideline (if not already adopted) and audit against it.

One very good example of a national guideline worthy of consideration (and is on the verge of becoming a national diktat) is the National Service Framework (NSF) standard for screening for diabetic retinopathy. Diabetic retinopathy is the most common cause of blindness in working-age people in the UK. Although potentially 50 per cent of those who develop proliferative diabetic retinopathy will lose their sight within 2 years, early detection of this condition coupled with treatment can halve the risk of sight loss. According to recommendations, all people diagnosed with diabetes should be offered diabetic retinopathy screening.

It may be seen, therefore, that the consideration of national guidelines often leads to the awareness of standards, and the need to audit against them.

Local guideline, process or committee

It is good practice to perpetually audit against local guidelines and standards. Many of these standards may also be national guidelines. Several local boards and committees are vital for standards, and may provide first-rate ammunition for clinical audit. Although the topic of adverse events (see above) should technically be included in this category (as a local process and committee), we the authors feel that its segregation as an independent paragraph is a measure of its importance. A very important additional example of a local process is 'patient outcome monitoring'. This may include formal complaints and patients' experience trackers.

It is vital that 'auditable items' are included in the agenda of these boards and committees and that these are in turn fed into the clinical audit committee for registration.

The trust may view these important local processes as key to operational success, and may therefore mandate audit projects to chart progress; these therefore develop into 'local diktats' (see below).

Local diktat

The trust may attach sufficient importance to a national or local guideline, and therefore insist on a relevant audit, via the clinical audit department. As described above, awareness of a national guideline may be a prompt for clinical audit in order to achieve quality, whereas local guidelines and processes may trigger a mandatory audit to maximise operational performance. An example of a departmental process/guideline/protocol commonly converted into a local diktat is perhaps a hygiene policy, where implementation may lead to the demonstration of the achievement of quality to third parties (for example the Care Quality Commission.)

Key points

- Triggers: focus the mind; identify reasons for projects; demonstrate the path to quality

- Perception as a trigger: recurrent clinical problems; feedback; direct observation

- Adverse events are potent triggers

- National Guidelines: these may originate from a learned society or any other body. Increasingly, trusts are proactively seeking to capture high profile national guidelines and auditing against them if they are relevant to practice

- National diktat: a mandatory audit may be required from a national authoritative body

- Local guideline, process or committee: it is good practice to audit against local standards within a rolling programme. Many local processes and committees are vital for standards, and may provide ammunition for clinical audit

- Local diktat: the trust attaches sufficient importance to a national or local guideline, and makes the audit against this standard mandatory

References

Department of Health, (2000) *An organisation with a memory: Report of an expert group on learning from adverse events in the NHS*, The Stationery Office, London.

Patient Safety Observatory, (2007) Executive Summary: *Slips, trips and falls in hospital*, National Patient Safety Agency, London.

Chapter 5 Embarking on a clinical audit

Issues to consider when identifying the audit topic

There are many audit tools that are available to help to prioritise and select appropriate topics for audit. These may include scoring systems which rank topics in order of importance. For example quality impact analyses and locally developed grids may list selection criteria and rank topics according to local priorities. In practice it is far commoner (and cheaper), however, for doctors to analyse vital criteria and commence on the basis of these.

Impact

The importance of the identification of a trigger for clinical audit has already been discussed. The actual selection of the topic may be more targeted when the areas of impact are examined. These may include:

- Personal practice: for example, a radiologist may assess his or her consistency of standards by requesting colleagues to re-issue his or her reports (assuming that their reports are seen as 'the standard')

- Local practice

- Regional/national practice: audits of regional or national practice are often mandatory, and will have been incorporated into the local hospital audit committee plan (see 'National diktat', Chapter 4).

Risk, volume and cost

High risk

Important attention must be drawn to procedures or clinical services that could potentially lead to harm to patients and/or healthcare professionals. Projects evaluating clinical practice are therefore crucial. This may be derived from the trust's 'risk register.' Indeed, the trigger may have been an adverse event (see 'Adverse event (and near miss)', Chapter 4.) Needle-stick injury is a well known example.

High volume

A high volume of procedures or patients demands the design of a good clinical audit to determine the smooth running of the activity. These activities or procedures are more prone to errors and therefore demand vigilance. An appropriate example may be the use of plain radiographs, where simple errors such as mislabelling of images or imaging the wrong person need to be addressed.

High cost

This receives attention, as the inappropriate use of an expensive test or treatment may lead to unnecessarily high expenditure. Therefore appropriate indications should be developed for these interventions and ensuing clinical audits may be conducted to monitor adherence to the recommended indications.

As the National Institute for Health and Clinical Excellence (NICE) has been entrusted with responsibility to evaluate the cost-effectiveness of an intervention, and make recommendations for its use, these recommendations may on occasions serve as standards.

Other considerations for defining the audit topic

It should be remembered that topics with one or more of the

above characteristics may not automatically be ideal for selection. The following questions may address some other areas that need consideration:

- Is there wide variation in practice?

- Is there local concern about a practice?

- Are standards/guidelines available? If not, is there a consensus on good clinical practice?

- Is the topic a priority for the local department or organisation?

- Is it practical to undertake the audit?

- Is information easy to obtain for the audit?

- Can changes be made for the audited problem?

- Who needs to be involved in ensure the implementation of changes?

Defining the aims

After identifying the topic, objectives should be clearly defined and the aims put in place to maintain the correct direction of the audit. This allows for better selection of methodology for data collection and analysis. Examples of clear and concise aims are:

- To ensure that a certain patient population is seen within a definite timeline in the appropriate clinic

- To improve the service delivery of a certain new procedure or intervention

- To increase the cost-effectiveness of a particular service provision

Defining the criteria

For a clinical audit project to run smoothly, it is vital that there is an explicit statement describing an area of care being measured. Some aspects to consider are included here.

Characteristics of good criteria: specific, measurable and achievable

Criteria need to be specific to an area of care or outcome. An ambiguous criterion is confusing, ast the auditors may have problems in data acquisition.

There should be elements of care that can be measured objectively. The question of 'what can be measured' is dealt with elegantly in Donabedian's (1988) quality model for measurable criteria. For example, even subjective topics such as patient satisfaction may be addressed with a satisfaction scale to enable objective measurement. This allows good information collation and analysis.

From a practical and realistic viewpoint, the criteria have to be achievable. It should be understood that each department and hospital is different, and that criteria that are achievable in one location may not be in another.

Types of criteria: structure, process and outcome

Donabedian's quality model mentioned above sets out three distinct areas: structure, process and outcome. It is common for projects to touch all three aspects simultaneously.

Criteria for structure may be interpreted as items required for clinical practice. This may involve the provision of equipment and physical space, the number of staff and the appropriate skill mix, as well as organisational arrangements. An example could include the provision of an out-of-hours imaging service (which clearly must incorporate sufficiently skilled staff and doctors).

Criteria based on process refer to the decisions and actions taken by healthcare professionals. They may involve communication with patients, investigations, treatments, interventional procedures and documentation.

Criteria may be based on the outcome following healthcare interventions. Examples include health status, level of knowledge or patient satisfaction. A good example of a commonly audited topic is that of blood pressure control in a specific patient population, such as patients with diabetes.

Defining the gold standards

One definition of a clinical standard is the level of care that must be achieved for any particular criterion (Irvine and Irvine 1991), and is usually expressed as a percentage. In all cases, the standards set for the criteria have to be practical and realistic in a given local environment. In addition the standard used needs to reflect the importance of the criterion, both clinically and in relation to any medico-legal consequences. The standard has also been defined as 'the percentage of events that should comply with the criterion' (Baker and Fraser 1995). It is against the standard and criterion that your own audit outcomes will be measured and compared.

When setting standards it would be appropriate to consider the resources of your department in relation to a variety of parameters, including financial resources, personnel, facilities available, the likelihood of patient compliance and demographics. The method and type of standard set depend very much on the aims of the audit project. If the aim is to achieve a level of performance just above that which is currently set, this is referred to as a 'stretch standard'. In contrast a 'nominative standard' is one that is determined on comparing performance with other members (individuals or group) participating in the audit.

Additional categories for guidance include:

- Minimum standard: this is the lowest acceptable standard of performance; minimum standards are often used to distinguish acceptable and unacceptable clinical practice

- Ideal standard: this describes the care possible under ideal conditions, with no constraint. Such a standard implies that criteria must be met in all conditions

- Optimum standard: this is the standard lying between 'minimum' and 'ideal'. Setting an optimum standard is often the most realistic and practical option. This requires judgement, discussion and consensus among other team members.

It is possible to audit against minimum, ideal and optimum standards concurrently in one project. The findings of such a project may for example demonstrate that minimum standards are met, yet optimum and ideal standards are not.

Data can normally be categorised into three groups:

1. Those which conform to the criteria

2. Those which do not conform, but fit the exceptions

3. Those which do not conform to the criteria

Using evidence base to identify a standard

It is essential to invest sufficient time in order to review published research related to the topic, to help define the audit standard. In most cases much of this process can be done using national databases (Cochrane and Athens being among the most commonly used in the UK.) As mentioned in Chapter 2, some high profile topics have already accrued national clinical guidelines through National Service Frameworks.

Situations however can and do arise where, even after doing a thorough literature search, only poor research-based evidence exists for the chosen audit topic. Where this occurs, and the topic is nevertheless considered vital, other methods of evidence should be taken into consideration. This may take the shape of a general consensus of opinion published from a multidisciplinary panel of experts, or patient preferences outlined by the use of questionnaires or surveys. When there is a wealth of literature at your disposal, the challenge is to find standards which are the most relevant. When there is a genuine absence of objective evidence to aid the identification of standards, one may consider manufacturing one that is credible and locally applicable.

Target population, timeframe and venue

One must decide early on in the project on the target population to be audited. (This is dealt with in more detail in Chapter 6, Acquisition, interpretation and analysis of data.) If a target population is large (for example all hypertensives), systematic or random sampling may be instituted. The timing of sampling is also vital, as discrepancies may occur in different seasons and different years. The site of data sampling may be influential, for example in projects dealing with the management of tuberculosis. Therefore, whether carrying out a retrospective or a prospective analysis, it is appropriate to decide on the target population, timeframe and venue.

Clinical audit framework

An audit project needs to have a framework in order to improve and maintain its quality, and facilitate organisation. Three important aspects are quality assurance, funding and timeline.

Quality assurance

All clinical audit projects without exception should facilitate improved quality assurance. This provides an overarching aim for each project, and hopefully prevents them from developing into 'tick-box exercises'. Each NHS organisation has the responsibility of ensuring that quality is maintained and improved in consequence to every clinical audit project, and therefore a robust clinical audit assessment framework may be developed and utilised by these organisations as a tool for quality assurance. Walshe and Spurgeon (1997), from the University of Birmingham, suggested a framework that included nine elements:

1. Reasons for topic selection (triggers and criteria)

2. Impact

3. Costs

4. Objectives

5. Involvement

6. Use of evidence

7. Project management

8. Methods

9. Evaluation

In addition to these, ethical issues should also be considered, although most clinical audits do not need ethical approval.

Funding and expenses

(See also our section 'Funding for projects', Chapter 3.) Funding is a crucial part of a clinical audit. Many healthcare professionals tend to underestimate the role of funding in running an audit project. If projects are expensive, their costs must be justifiable. Full or part time clinical audit department staff with expertise also cost money, as does ring-fenced participation time for clinical staff.

Many clinical audit projects have cost effectiveness implications. For example, if an audit project can identify inefficiencies in a service, the consequent service improvement may lead to improved cost-effectiveness. Therefore, the cost of running the project may be offset against the proposed savings. The opposite can also occur, however. A successful project may uncover deficiencies in certain aspects of clinical care and changes may lead to increased expense. It is vital that when planning such projects, the possible increase in expenditure is incorporated into the budget planning.

Timeline

Time issues are usually one of the biggest obstacles in completing an audit. It is also a reason for abandonment of a clinical audit. The best way to tackle this problem is to allocate protected time to investigate the topic for audit, and to collect and analyse data. All staff involved in the audit need to understand and be committed to allocating time to participate fully. The clinical audit department also needs to be realistic if a project is clearly stalling, and has taken an inordinate amount of time with little progress. On these occasions the auditors may need to be given time limits and ultimatums.

Identification of potential barriers to implementation

The issue of implementation will be dealt with in Chapter 8. It is important to recognise at this stage that even if the clinical audit project is well conducted and the deficits are well demarcated, the subsequent implementation process may be doomed to fail if potential barriers are not identified in a timely fashion. Two typical examples are worth considering:

- Post audit, there may still be a lack of change in behaviour. This may be a consequence of either a lack of interest in some individuals, or the perception amongst some individuals that performance is good, and that therefore change is unnecessary.

- During the implementation process, despite the creation of high quality guidelines, it is not uncommon for the latter not to be followed. This may be a consequence of either a perception amongst some individuals that they lack knowledge, or denial, where perhaps the guideline is not considered reputable.

Knowledge of these barriers will not only help mould the implementation process in the future, but will also improve understanding in this preparation stage.

The clinical audit team and other key individuals

Clinical audit is an exercise in teamwork involving a multitude of people, ranging from clinical to non-clinical staff. They are all stakeholders, and will very likely benefit from being involved in the project. Most projects cannot be managed single-handedly, as they need different skills at different stages of the process. The approach therefore needs the sharing of methods and results among the multidisciplinary teams. This commendable aim is not, however, easily achieved.

Boundaries and interfaces should be examined, joined and crossed, far beyond those normally described in relation to the frequently-used term 'multidisciplinary team'.

Good examples of working across interfaces include:

- Primary and secondary care

- Clinicians and management

- Healthcare professionals and patients. Patients have not historically been used in project teams as often as they should. They are the ultimate stakeholders and the ultimate end-users, and as such are able to provide invaluable insight into most topics.

Management and leadership both play an important role in clinical audit, as they do in other quality improvement projects. In this respect both healthcare and clinical audit depend on the quality of teamwork, and the teams themselves. It may be argued that more emphasis should be given to the development of team leadership and other such skills. Enabling improvement in quality through clinical audit frequently depends on constructing and managing relationships as well as resources across the organisation as a whole. It is important to have people who are approachable and willing to address concerns within the audit team. Many NHS trusts provide training on a wide variety of quality improvement skills, often primarily targeting hospital managers, clinicians and those involved in clinical governance.

There are many other types of skills and expertise needed, and they may be categorised broadly into themes. By understanding the type of skills needed, one will be in a position to invite appropriate people into the clinical audit team.

1. Information and knowledge support: the gathering of information through an established source is often best done with the help of staff from the library, while access to information technology (IT) may be achieved through IT personnel.

2. Data management: there should be sufficient knowledge among the team members to enable adequate data collection, collation, analysis and presentation.

3. Facilitation: an audit team involving many members must be facilitated by the lead auditor to ensure smooth running of the group.

4. Project management: this is important in all types of projects. Every project needs to be well managed in order to progress smoothly. This may also be achieved by the lead auditor.

5. Training: clinical audit staff have an important role to play in training some or all of the team members during the project

After addressing the skills needed for a successful clinical audit, one should quickly identify the people needed for the project, and the team members may include:

*   Clinical and non-clinical staff providing the skills described above

*   Service users (this may include patients, as highlighted above)

*   People whose support may be required to implement the changes in practice

Fortunately, most NHS organisations have a clinical audit department to facilitate projects. As described in Chapter 2, the clinical audit department may provide advice about existing projects, provide information on data collection and analysis, and facilitate presentation.

The clinical audit project will carry more meaning if the team dynamics encourage a motivating environment, in order to allow all the auditors to remain committed and develop the desire to sustain and improve the level of performance in their particular healthcare field. The aim is for an environment in which all members, both junior and senior, feel comfortable about approaching others to share ideas, concerns, and discuss individual and group objectives. This is most easily done by organising regular group meetings to achieve the objectives outlined.

In a large organisation it is not always possible or feasible for any one individual to deal with everyone's concerns, even if he or she is the lead auditor. While providing input and having the final say on controversial or grey areas, the lead auditor should be regarded as a member who can be approached by all involved staff. This person may choose to delegate areas of responsibility to others. He or she should also be able to inspire confidence, have the desire and the necessary skills to initiate the process of change, and help promote an environment in which such a change will be welcomed by those affected. It is not paramount to be present throughout the whole process, but he or she should play a pivotal role in starting the audit and help to create a sense of unity or common purpose. Strong leadership should not be underestimated. It is not uncommon for interest amongst auditors to wane once the initial novelty of the audit 'experience' has worn off. The lead auditor may play a fundamental role here to maintain motivation, focus on goals and continue the drive for implementation.

Where projects have a strong relationship to national standards, it is not uncommon to have an individual well versed in management to take the role of project lead, or some fundamental role in the audit process; the participation of managers should therefore be actively encouraged.

It can sometimes prove difficult to obtain the physical involvement of all the relevant key players at all times in the audit process. The most common reason sited is the lack of available time. Some may regard clinical audit project meetings as yet another activity taking clinicians away from their clinical commitments. However, it is essential that clinical audit is given the importance and respect afforded to (for example) medical education.

Clinical audit (ethics) governance

Although clinical audit projects do not usually require ethics approval, at times this may be unclear. The most important rule is that clinical audit should always be conducted within an ethical framework. This rule has a large impact on the way that a clinical audit is devised, and essentially implies that patients' confidentiality must be maintained at all times, abiding by the principles of the Data Protection Act.

All audit projects must comply with some general standards:

- Only the minimum amount of patient-identifiable information should be collected

- The data should be anonymised as early on in the project as possible

- The appropriate security measures should be taken to keep patient information secure and available only to those who need to know

- All identifiable data should be deleted once the final report has been produced and distributed

- No identifiable data must be included in the audit report or in any presentation of findings

A vital point to note is that none of the issues being audited should fall outside the realm of routine clinical management.

The audit team may on occasions include members who are not employees of the local organisation; examples include medical students or volunteers. These individuals should obtain an honorary contract if they need to access patients' notes and a member of the local organisation must take responsibility for how and where clinical information is accessed.

The clinical audit department, perhaps with the help of the research and development department, should be in a position to provide advice about the latest guidance on issues of ethics and patients' consent. They should also take shared responsibility for the following clinical audit governance issues:

- Ensuring that explicit consent is obtained where it is necessary under terms of the local policy

- Authorising the information leaflets and consent forms where explicit consent is required

- Authorising the arrangements for gathering and anonymising retrospective information where implied consent is relied on

Any doubts with regard to governance and ethics should always be clarified with the clinical audit department and the local trust Research and Development department (ethics committee).

Some specific additional issues are listed below:

1. Is the project 'audit' or 'research'?

The distinction between audit and research is not usually difficult.

- Will the project involve measuring practice against agreed or defined standards or guidelines?

- Does the project involve interventions which may be considered 'routine'?

- Does the project attempt to establish whether one intervention is superior to another?

Clearly one would answer in the affirmative for the first two questions for clinical audit projects, and the third for research projects.

There may be situations where the proposed project contains elements of both audit and research. In this case, formal ethics approval is required.

2. Is a patient survey planned?

Patient or user satisfaction surveys that do not contain any clinical information do not need ethics approval. However, even if the survey is an audit, there may be situations whereby an ethical dimension may arise, mainly involving patients' rights, dignity and time.

The ethical issues arising in a survey audit consist of ways of identifying patients for the audit, confidentiality of patients' responses and any disturbance caused to patients. The most important aspect is whether the survey interferes with the patient's treatment in any way. Patients are occasionally fearful that by being asked questions about their treatment and care, they might subsequently receive a change in treatment and care plans. They should be reassured to the contrary. One should always refer to the local trust Research and Development department (ethics committee) for further advice when deciding about the need for ethics approval.

3. Is publication planned?

The main issue in publication of the audit is whether the topic, methodology and results may be generalised beyond the local audience and setting. If generalisation is the case, it is normally good practice to request consideration of publication by the local trust ethics committee. Some journal editors will not publish clinical audit articles unless ethics approval has been sought. It is useful in these situations to have already obtained a supporting letter from the ethics committee stating its position on ethics approval.

4. Are all team members bound by a duty of confidentiality?

All team members participating in the clinical audit project need to understand and adhere to all necessary steps to safeguard patients' confidentiality. The act of data collection has several ethical implications for those involved in its implementation. Confidentiality is achieved by protecting the identity of patients, carers, guardians, clinical staff and any other members involved in the information gathering process. At the time of presentation none of these individuals should be identifiable by name, hospital number, ward or bed allocation, or any other means that could expose their identity. In the earlier stages of the project, identifiable personal health information about patients should not be disclosed to anyone who does not provide direct patient care. There must also be full anonymity in the audit database.

The collected information must be sufficient for the purpose of the audit. Collecting additional irrelevant information contravenes the Data Protection Act. Finally, data should not be held longer than necessary. Completed audit data collection forms should be destroyed once the data have been completed and action plans recommended.

An example of the relevance of anonymisation of clinical staff may be found in projects dealing with individual performance. In these circumstances extreme care must be taken to group or categorise participants when their anonymity could be threatened. For example, in a group of surgeons being audited for their infection rates, there may only be one orthopaedic surgeon, a few plastic surgeons, a few ENT (ear, nose and throat) surgeons and several general surgeons. In such a scenario it would seem prudent to group the orthopaedic, plastic and ENT surgeons, taking care not to reveal their identity by stating which procedures had been performed.

There is a considerable body of information from professional organisations relating to the issue of data protection. Those involved in the audit process should be familiar with the Data Protection Act 1998, and the issues therein pertaining to patient confidentiality. Another useful source of knowledge on this topic is available from the General Medical Council (GMC), in the booklet, *Confidentiality: Protecting and providing information* (2004); in particular, paragraphs 13–15 pertain to clinical audit.

5. Do I need patients' consent?

Consent may be a delicate issue from time to time. The ideal rule is that in all cases, patients' consent should be obtained at all times to fulfil the criteria for patients' rights. Unfortunately, this may not be practical for all types of audits. McKinney et al. (2005) demonstrated that systematically obtaining individual signed consent for sharing patient identifiable information with an externally located clinical audit database is difficult. The need for every single clinical audit project to obtain individual signed consent from the patient or the healthcare provider may deter healthcare professionals from conducting many projects. Some guidance is therefore provided below.

The Data Protection Act 1998 (already mentioned), the Human Rights Act 1998, the Common Law Duty of Confidentiality and the principles established by the Caldicott Committee all protect the privacy of patients and their information.

Consent for the use of information

Under the Common Law Duty of Confidentiality the use and processing of confidential patient information may occur only with the patient's consent. Legislation allows consent to be assumed (implied consent) or actively obtained (explicit consent).

Situations for explicit consent, whereby patients' consent must be actively sought, are:

- If there is a possibility that an individual will be affected by any aspect of the project, including personal involvement, subsequent contact or feedback of information

- If it is practical to approach individuals to obtain their explicit consent

- Where personal information may be disclosed to a third party organisation.

The most frequent types of audit work that require explicit consent are:

- Patient questionnaires

- Observed practice.

Explicit patients' consent is not necessary when a study or audit can be carried out without using or accessing confidential identifiable patients' data at any stage. On occasions explicit consent may not be required even when it is necessary to obtain identifiable information for the audit project, if the use of patient data is for the provision of care and clinical audit and is effectively a condition of receiving treatment. In these situations the acceptance of treatment by the patient implies consent for the audit.

There are some criteria that must be fulfilled in the situation of implied consent from patients:

1. Patients involved in the audit will receive information about the use to which their details are put

2. Formal healthcare records are used

3. The project does not affect the clinical care of patients directly

4. The data is gathered and anonymised by a member of the healthcare team

Gaining patients' consent

Once it has been established that a clinical audit needs patient consent, relevant information must be disseminated to patients about the audit in which they are involved. An information leaflet may be a convenient method to do this. Certain information should be listed in the leaflet as detailed below:

- The identity of the NHS organisation as the data controller and the initial recipient of the information

- A list of organisations to which the anonymised personal data may be disclosed

- The purpose and methodology of the project, including a basic explanation of what information is involved and a description of the benefits that may result from the project

- How any information disclosed will be used and a guarantee that results will be presented anonymously

- How the information will be protected and assured, including the duration for which the information will be retained and under what circumstances it will be destroyed

- The identities of participating organisations

- Contacts for raising queries about the project

- Contacts for raising queries relating to data protection or confidentiality within the NHS organisation

- Information about the right to decline participation (and an associated guarantee that the refusal will subsequently have no adverse affect on treatment).

The information leaflet provided must allow for disabilities, illiteracy, diverse cultural conditions and language differences.

Once the patient has sufficient information about the audit, a written consent may be obtained. The patient consent form must include the following:

- Title and reference of the project

- The name of the project lead

- Reference to the information leaflet

The written consent is valid only for the project specified in the consent form. All signed consent forms should be retained and filed with the medical record when the project is completed.

When seeking written consent from patients, they should be provided with:

- Honest, clear, objective information about the data usage and their choices

- An opportunity for patients to talk to someone whom they can trust and of whom they can ask questions

- Reasonable time and privacy to reach decisions

- Support and explanation about any form that they may need to sign

- A choice as to whether to be contacted in the future about further uses for the project findings, and how the contact should be made.

These points offer a firm basis for obtaining consent from patients for an audit project. Each consent form needs to be tailored to the specific audit topic and the target population. However, the most important issue is that patients be given sufficient information and reassurance about confidentiality, as well as the opportunity for any queries to be made.

Registration of the audit proposal with the clinical audit department

It is vital that the clinical audit department is involved for the entirety of the clinical audit project, and that every new project should be registered. Only in this way can the department become a comprehensive source of information with regard to clinical audit and audit projects for those inside and outside the trust. Involvement of the department will also enable their members to provide guidance and help in the early stages of planning. The clinical audit department may be a source of audit topic selection, as it will have a list of existing and recently completed audit topics. Furthermore, the department may advise on the support that can be provided in terms of data collection and acquiring medical notes. Some larger clinical audit departments are also in a position to provide assistance in statistical analysis.

The registration form should ideally identify at the outset all significant issues about the project from design to ethics, consent, data collection and implementation. At this point, the clinical audit department will have the opportunity to advise on issues that may be conflicting and inappropriate for the local setting.

Figure 5.1 is a common pathway from project lead contact to commencement. Each organisation will have variations in this pathway to accommodate local requirements and priorities.

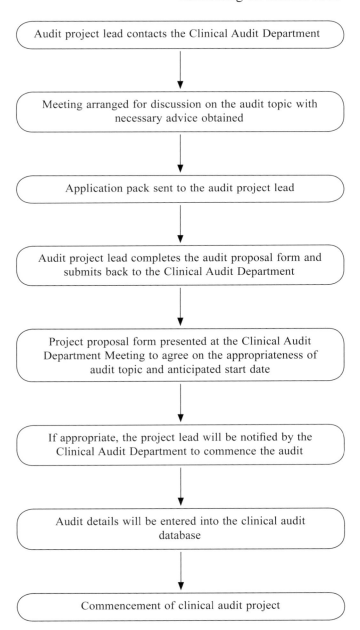

Figure 5.1   Clinical audit proposal pathway

Key points

- Issues to consider when identifying the audit topic: impact, risk, volume and cost

- Define the aims

- Define the criteria: characteristics and types

- Define gold standards: if possible, use evidence-based practice

- Consider target population, timeframe and venue

- Clinical audit framework: quality assurance, funding, timeline

- Identify individuals who should be involved: be inclusive and consider crossing traditional boundaries

- Ethics and governance: confidentiality and consent

- Registration and involvement of the clinical audit department

References

Baker R; Fraser RC; *Development of review criteria: linking guidelines and assessment of quality.* BMJ 1995 Aug 5;311 (7001): 370 – 373. Eli Lilly National Clinical Audit Centre, Department of General Practice, University of Leicester

Donabedian A (1998.) The *quality of care. How can it be assessed? JAMA* **260**:1743–8.

GMC, *Confidentiality: Protecting and providing information* (2004). A GMC publication. In particular, paragraphs 13–15 pertain to clinical audit. A electronic version is available at www.gmc-uk.org.

Irvine D, Irvine S. (1991) *Making Sense of Audit*, Radcliffe Medical Press, Oxford.

McKinney PA, Jones S, Parslow R *et al.* (2005) for the PICANet Consent

Study Group. *A feasibility study of signed consent for the collection of patient identifiable information for a national paediatric clinical audit database. BMJ*; **330**:877–9.

Walshe K, Spurgeon P. (1997) *Clinical Audit Assessment Framework: Audit project detailed assessment and improvement plan*. Health Services Management Centre, University of Birmingham and NHS Executive. Birmingham.

Further reading

Health Informatics Unit (2007) *Generic Medical Record-keeping Standards*. Royal College of Physicians, London.

Chapter 6 Acquisition, interpretation and analysis of data

Having set the topic, criteria, standard and aims, one must turn to the often arduous task of collecting the data in order to produce an effective and worthwhile audit. A means of collecting the data-set needs to be identified, even if there is a wealth of resources available.

The outcome of any audit process is only as meaningful as the sum of the quantitative and qualitative parts identified in the data accumulated. Where does one start? At the outset the audit lead should have some idea of the strengths and weaknesses of the team members. These skills need to be utilised so that each member of the team is able to work constructively and within their capabilities to help achieve the common goal. Some members may, for example, be skilled at mathematical calculation, while others may have a particular aptitude for using information technology systems to design charts and developing database systems. Some may be more confident in their ability to analyse and report findings and express this in high quality prose.

Data collection – general principles

It is imperative that the team involved all have some interest in the topic being audited and the same goal in mind, namely to look for methods and ways in which to improve practice. This enthusiasm will drive the project. Throughout the audit process individual team members should act as a source of encouragement, particularly to the less experienced individuals involved. Junior doctors with short attachments to the trust should be reassured that if they are inevitably involved in only part of the data collection, this contribution to clinical audit will be recognised.

Especially in handwritten clinical notes, there may be difficulties with interpretation. It is expected that different individuals will interpret data in different ways. For example, an entry of 'Temp' followed by a cross may be interpreted as suggesting that no temperature had been recorded by one auditor, whereas a colleague, on seeing the same entry, may interpret this to mean that the temperature had been recorded but was abnormal. To avoid such potential problems it will be essential to have clear explicit data extraction guidelines before starting this process. On doing this, the reliability of two or more individuals involved in the process can be assessed using sample data to see whether there is consistency.

When some information is not immediately apparent, there may be differences in thoroughness. One individual may sift through different volumes and sections to find the data required, whereas another may have a lower threshold for regarding the information as missing and therefore spend less time and effort to find it.

Who should collect the data?

Data collection and analysis can be very time-consuming in everyday practice. Typically all the auditors are closely involved in the data collection process. However, as described above, different roles may be ascribed to different individuals with appropriate skills, and complete involvement may not be possible for some junior doctors whose attachment to a trust may be shorter than the time required to complete data acquisition. The clinical audit department may on occasions be called upon if appropriate to participate in the data collection process.

Methods of data collection

Data collection needs to be performed in accordance with the purpose and criteria of the audit. A number of common methods are employed, with arguably the most common being the use of patients' case notes and clinical records. Here, perhaps more than elsewhere, careful meticulous technique is required to ensure that data are obtained in a consistent fashion and bias is avoided. The advantage of having a pre-designed tick-box pro forma is that data can be more easily and speedily quantified. In this way, future audits on the same topic can also be performed in a more efficient manner. The pro forma should contain all the relevant outcome measures from the outset.

Information to include in the pro forma

This obviously depends on the topic being audited; however, there are some general points to consider when designing the pro forma:

- It should be typewritten with clear instructions on how to complete the form and where to return it

- It may be appropriate to include the name and contact details of the audit lead

- The form should be titled and dated

- Each patient's identity must be protected; this may be coded. To enable the auditors to return to case notes and review data, it would be appropriate to have a separate record, listing the code numbers correlating with the patients' hospital numbers. Clearly, this separate record should be destroyed at an appropriate time

- All data should be stored safely as according to the recommendations of the Data Protection Act

- Health professionals must also have their anonymity protected

An example of an audit pro forma (used for collecting information on infection rates on a surgical ward) is shown in Figure 6.1.

INFECTION PRO-FORMA

Name: _____

Age: _____

Hosp: I.D _____

Admission Date: _____

Discharge Date: _____

Internal PT ☐   External referral ☐

Emergency ☐   Elective ☐

Hospital admission: critical care ☐   High dependency ☐   Ward ☐

Diagnosis: _____

Name of operative procedure : _____

_____

Length of procedure : _____

Date of procedure: _____

Surgeon status: _____

Consultant ☐   Staff grade ☐   Registrar ☐   SHO ☐

Date infection identified: _____

Name of infection isolated: _____

MRSA ☐   Clostridium difficile ☐

Other, specify ☐ _____

Isolate: _____

Sputum ☐   Blood ☐   Urine ☐   Stool ☐

CSF ☐   Localised wound ☐

Other, specify ☐ _____

Intra op antibiotic(s) used & mode _____

Post OP antibiotic(s) used, mode (per oral, intravenous, intrathecal) and duration:

_____

_____

Co-morbidity, if so state: _____

_____

Mortality: No ☐   Yes ☐

Figure 6.1   Data collection pro forma – infection rates

Targeting the sample population and methods of sampling

It is imperative at a very early stage to decide on the target population to be audited. Although the topic is included in this 'data' chapter, it is clear that the decisions with regard to targeting and sampling should take place during the time of project conception.

Where the target population is particularly large, a sample of this would need to be extracted and audited. If, for example, the aim is to audit the management of hypertension in a district general hospital (DGH), it is likely that this would be too large an undertaking in itself. However, it may be a more practical and feasible option to audit the management of hypertension in a specific ward over a 3-month period. By taking an appropriate subset of the population, the expectation is that generalisation will be possible, and that the results would give a good indication for those expected of the whole population. As an alternative, by taking a random sample of patients, one could also hope to achieve a representative result. Such random sampling may be carried out with the help of most statistical textbooks and a random numbers table, or alternatively using mathematical computer software.

Where random sampling is not a viable option, systematic samples can be employed. This technique involves the selection of units from an ordered sampling frame. For example if bookshop owners wanted to observe the buying habits of their customers, by using systematic sampling, they could choose every fifth or tenth customer entering the shop and conduct the study on this sample. However, if the audit is associated with a smaller population size, e.g. patients with pancreatic malignancy on the general surgical wards, it may well be possible to collect the relevant data from the complete population and, in so doing, provide an insight into a truer performance. A common example of sampling in use is at the time of an election. Here opinion polls are commonly constructed in an effort to select samples that are indicative of the population as a whole.

The timing of sampling is critical. If a defined time period is not stated, there may be a huge discrepancy between the numbers and characteristics of patients involved during one set defined period compared with what you may expect at a different time of year. For example, if the prospective audit were based on the management and treatment of patients in a hospital presenting with pneumonia, you may be more likely to achieve a higher population over the winter months compared with what one would expect over summer. The site of data sampling should also be considered. If, for example, the aim is to audit the presentation and management of tuberculosis, geographical variation in numbers should not be overlooked before starting the project. It would be wise to compare the findings with those in different regions in order to provide a sense of the associated variation. Hence, whether carrying out a retrospective or a prospective analysis, it is usually appropriate to decide on a timeframe over which the data collection should be performed. An alternative strategy is to decide in advance that the data collection will stop when a specific minimum target number has been reached. One should bear in mind that larger patient numbers tend to be associated with a higher likelihood of achieving statistical significance.

Retrospective and prospective data collection

Retrospective data collection gives information about a clinical situation at a point in time in the past, depending on which period is covered. The main practical advantage is that the data collection can be carried out at a rate determined by the auditors, invariably faster than a prospective data collection. Auditors need to be wary that they may come across missing documentation and this needs to be investigated to make the collection complete. In contrast, a prospective collection will be for a predetermined period according to the audit requirements and so may take up more time at this initial stage of the audit project. The information provided prospectively is generally more useful at analysing the current level of performance, allowing the team to distinguish what needs to be done at present to maintain and improve quality.

Internal and external data acquisition

This descriptor simply identifies whether the organisation's data is acquired using individuals from within ('internal') or outside ('external') the organisation itself. The knowledge of external collectors, who may be able to approach the audit from a different viewpoint, is often important for the planning process. Internal acquisition is by far the commoner process.

Where external data collection is applied (more commonly performed when a national clinical audit is undertaken) external auditors usually require access to clinical case notes or the hospital's information technology (IT) systems. Therefore introducing them in a timely fashion to key members of clinical and management staff will help speed up and further the data collection.

Qualitative and quantitative data

Where data collection is predominantly in the form of descriptive text, for example patients' comments on a written or oral interview, or questionnaire, the collection is termed 'qualitative data'. Where possible it is easier to assimilate these data when they are clearly grouped in certain categories. For example, if patients are asked to rate how satisfactorily their blood pressure is controlled with a specific antihypertensive regimen, specific available options such as 'very good', 'good', 'satisfactory', 'poor' and 'very poor', facilitate an easier analysing tool.

In contrast, quantitative data tends to be numerical; this appears to be the predominant form of data used in clinical audit.

Table 6.1 describes some of the more commonly used terms.

Criterion: A measurable unit derived from the aims and objectives for carrying out each instruction. Criteria are often divided into those that are clinical, hence directly related to patient care, or organisational, so targeted towards the organisation providing that care.

Settings: The environment on which the criterion is based. This can include the type of NHS organisation e.g. district general hospital, tertiary centre, primary care trust etc, or it can relate the level of health care.

Exceptions: These should be made clear from the outset. They concern those members or parts of the organisation where strict adherence to the guidelines suggested may not be appropriate.

Standard: A minimum level of acceptable performance for a particular criterion. In most circumstances this is ideally set at 100% or 0%, it is usually recognised that this may initially be a difficult target to attain for most organisations.

Data source: The collection or areas where we would expect the data could be derived. This can vary at a local, regional or national level.

Structure: Namely the resources you have available. This includes current knowledge, skills and attitudes.

Result: Refers to the total that have met the audit standard. This can be given as an individual number, but is more commonly expressed as a percentage.

Outcome: This can imply the health benefits, cost-effectiveness or patient satisfaction.

Audit cycle: Clinical audit is best regarded as a continuous cycle of improvement, the process commonly shown as a cyclical diagram beginning with the identification of a problem or objective to the final stage comprising re-audit to assess the impact of the implemented changes.

Table 6.1   Description of some of the more common terms used in clinical audit

The role of information technology

Once the data has been collected and all the pro formas completed, the information should ideally be organised into a format that allows for ease of analysis. This may be integrated into a spreadsheet (more suitable for quantitative data), or database (also caters for qualitative data). Numerous programs exist to allow the data to be displayed on these packages. The nature of the software package is not important, provided it is practical and functional. A clinical audit study in colorectal cancer by Ugolini *et al.* (2009) suggests the need for, and confirms the usefulness of, a dedicated database in surgical audit activity.

Many hospital trusts have computerised patient records, which often allow the data collection process to run more smoothly.

Data interpretation

Depending on the nature of the audit it may be appropriate to compare existing data with results from a previous audit (on the same subject), against the expected or ideal outcome, and possibly also a comparison of one unit's findings with another. When interpreting these comparisons the usual considerations should be made:

- Differences in financial input

- The grade and numbers of staff

- The size of the unit/department

- The size of the population served

Data analysis

After tabulation of data into a spreadsheet and/or database, the findings need to be efficiently described. This may be achieved by displaying the data using tables or charts.

Pie charts (Figure 6.2)

A pie chart is a circular chart, divided into regions or 'sectors'. In a pie chart, the area (or volume in a spherical three-dimensional model) of a sector is proportional to the quantity that it represents – the greater the associated area, the larger the frequency. In this way, pie charts are most useful in displaying nominal or ordinal data.

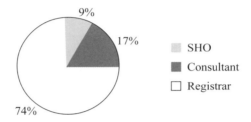

Figure 6.2   Grade of Surgeon Performing an Appendicectomy in a DGH over 1 year

Bar charts (Figure 6.3)

A bar chart is also very useful for displaying nominal or ordinal data. Here there are rectangular bars with lengths proportional

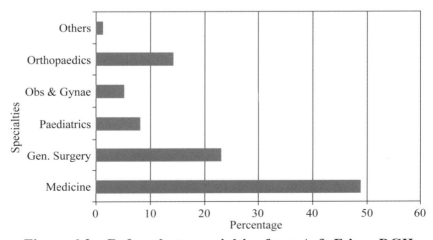

Figure 6.3   Referrals to specialties from A & E in a DGH over a four-month period

to the values that they represent. In this way they can be used to compare two or more values. The bars may be placed horizontally or vertically (the latter is more common). Gaps between the bars indicate that they are discrete entities.

Histograms (Figure 6.4)

These are graphical displays of tabulated frequencies shown as bars. They are suitable for displaying numerical data, and not appropriate for nominal or ordinal data. They demonstrate the proportion of cases falling into each of several categories. Histograms are particularly useful in analysing whether data are normally distributed, a normal distribution being one that is symmetrical and bell shaped with a peak at the mean.

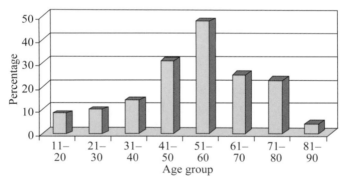

Figure 6.4   Histogram showing the ages of patients undergoing inguinal hernia repair in a Tertiary centre

Statistical application

You may wish to consider more detailed analysis of the data through the use of statistical methods to determine if the results could be regarded as 'significant'. For this to be the case, meticulous planning is required from the outset. The project design must allow for this, as must the patient numbers involved. Significance testing is particularly beneficial in reviewing whether changes implemented after the initial audit have produced results that can be regarded as statistically significant, and in this regard whether the change or changes to practice have been a worthwhile implementation.

Within a hospital trust, you will often find statistical expertise, perhaps contained within the research and development department. It may be that a particular member of your audit team has statistical and software skills. There are many commercial software systems available; it is important that those used are up-to-date and user-friendly.

Any statistical analysis tools used should ideally include descriptive statistics, bivariate statistics, prediction for numerical outcomes and prediction for identifying groups.

A basic working knowledge of statistics is recommended, even for those individuals not fundamentally involved in the data analysis. This will help to make sense of the results, and also assist during presentations when one may be asked to contribute to discussions with regard to interpretation of data.

Statistical significance

Statistical significance is a mathematical phenomenon used to determine, in response to a proposed hypothesis, whether the results of data obtained are due to a specific relationship or the consequence of chance. Different degrees of statistical significance exist, and are ascribed 'p' values. For example: '$p < 0.05$' implies that one may be 95% confident that the result did not occur by chance, whereas '$p < 0.01$' implies that one may be 99% confident that the result did not occur by chance.

Making sense of the results

The results need to be methodically reviewed. Although it may seem obvious, it is easy for auditors to inadvertently ignore the original question:

> *How do our results fare in relation to the question formulated at the start of this audit?*

For example, does this trust manage its head injury patients in accordance with the guidelines set out by NICE? How do we perform in relation to meeting the nationally agreed 2-week target rule for seeing patients with a suspicion of cancer referred from GPs? In this way we are able to determine the percentage or proportion of patients whose care is within the acceptable or gold standard criteria.

Hence, the importance of achieving results which have both value on interpretation and statistical significance cannot be overemphasised.

An indication of the final results often becomes increasingly obvious as the dataset is analysed, although this is not necessarily the case. It is only once the results of the audit is known and understood that recommendations for change can be made.

Key points

- Data collection, general principles: teamwork; be aware of the variety in interpretation of data and thoroughness amongst team members

- Team working is vital for collection of data

- Consider creating a proforma for data collection

- Target population and methods of sampling: the population may be sampled in full, or alternatively random or systematic samples may be taken

- Data collection may be retrospective or prospective

- Data may be internal, external, qualitative or quantitative

- The role of IT is vital

- Data analysis: be aware of various charts as vehicles of representation; be aware of statistical applications

- Make sense of the results

References

Ugolini G; Rosati G; Montroni I; *et al* (2009). *An easy-to-use solution for clinical audit in colorectal cancer surgery, Surgery* 145(1): 86-92. Department of General surgery, Emergency surgery and Organ Transplantation, University of Bologna, Italy.

Chapter 7 Presentation and publication

The skills needed for presentation are generic, widely-required and essential for survival in medical forums far outside the realms of clinical audit. The general advice in this chapter will therefore be relevant for many situations, and will be particularly pertinent to the more junior doctors.

Taking time to present your findings allows others to hear your work and suggestions for change. This will provide a forum in addition to the written medium to further facilitate the local integration of changes. Presentations are also more likely to enthuse, when compared to the simple written word.

Many audits flounder at this stage, as junior doctors may move on to their next job, or they may be constrained for time. It is vital therefore that time is ring-fenced for clinical audit presentations, and that facilities are provided to allow junior doctors to travel back to their previous trust to present their project. There are many forums and methods of presentation.

Local presentations

Most healthcare professionals are now very familiar with local audit presentation. It is usual for each directorate or division to set aside one half-day a month or 1 hour a week for clinical audit. This time is often used to look crudely at volume of work, morbidity and mortality. However, this is also an opportunity to present any audit projects that have been completed in the department since the last meeting.

Once the project is complete, the lead auditor and the most senior member of the team should be made aware; a meeting may then be arranged in order to discuss the findings.

Subsequently, it will be necessary to inform the directorate audit lead and/or the clinical audit department. Some trusts arrange for all their local presentations to take place in the trust-wide audit days, organised by the clinical audit committee. Others also run local audit through the directorates and divisions, often with the help of an assistant general manager designated for audit activities. Slots for presentations are offered therefore by the clinical audit manager or the assistant general manager respectively. The type of presentation (usually electronic slides) should be clarified. Once the date is known, this should be shared with all of the other auditors. The lead auditor and senior members of the group should arrange for group based preparations, particularly in order to deal with difficult questions.

Usually the oral presentation is short, and is followed by questions and answers. Often posters will also be required. One should pay close attention to any rules or timing for slides, which should be kept simple, clear and professional. Bleeps, pagers and mobile phones should be switched off, to avoid distraction and irritation for the audience.

The presentation should be focussed, and follow some simple guidelines:

- Focus your presentation on what you did, what you found and how this will change things locally

- Keep the background and science relatively basic

- Ensure that the standard is defined early on

- Provide comparison of your results with other comparable groups if appropriate

- Make sure that the recommendations are sensible and feasible

The question-and-answer session may be quite challenging. The questions often range wider than the presentation and will likely focus on how these changes can be implemented, what extra resources are required and whether funding is necessary. It is important that all the individuals in the project group (in particular the lead auditor and senior members) contribute at this stage.

National and international presentations

The clinical audit presentation has historically had a low profile in these forums when compared to its elder brother, research. This may partly be a result of the (clearly wrong) perception that the findings are not considered sufficiently important.

Most specialties and subspecialties have their own annual conference. Although international conferences are considered prestigious, they are often in a position to accept a larger number of abstracts. Other national medical bodies such as the Royal Colleges and other medical societies also hold regular conferences. The opportunities are publicised on relevant websites. Finally, multi-disciplinary healthcare bodies specialising in clinical audit (described Chapter 2) hold generic conferences focussing on topics such as quality of care, healthcare delivery and patient safety.

Senior members of the project group must be prepared to be a resource when more junior doctors seek advice with regard to national and international presentations. Particular attention must be paid to deadlines, which are inevitably very strict. With regard to deadlines, one should cater for differences in time zones and the higher chance of websites crashing owing to simultaneous last-minute submissions.

Most national and international conferences have websites that include a list of recent poster and platform presentations; this should help provide guidance for quality, and also prevent repetition. There are usually preliminary programmes for the conference where one can establish important themes that will be discussed; one may therefore identify whether the audit project fits within a declared theme.

The requirement to produce a short (for example 250- to 500-word) abstract is an exercise in clarity and brevity of writing. Usually abstracts are in English, but it is important to remember that they may not be judged by someone whose first language is English; it is therefore vital that plain language is used. One should closely follow the guidelines for the abstract, for example the inclusion of aims, objectives and the word count. Finally if the abstract is accepted, many conferences publish the abstracts in a journal supplement or on their website; this may be considered a minor publication.

The poster presentation

There are many ways of preparing a poster and they all have their own advantages and drawbacks. At the conference there will usually be a space allocated (often approximately one metre square). Although one can print individual A4 sheets and arrange them within the allocated space, the most common and professional way of preparing the poster is by using a computer slide software package and then having the poster printed professionally.

It is important to read through the audit project meticulously before starting the poster preparation. Careful consideration should be applied to the context and background to the study and any additional information that may be needed for this section of the poster. Time should be taken to organise the results into a logical order. It should be remembered that some results will be best demonstrated as graphs. The latter will reduce the word count and provide an effective pictorial demonstration of results.

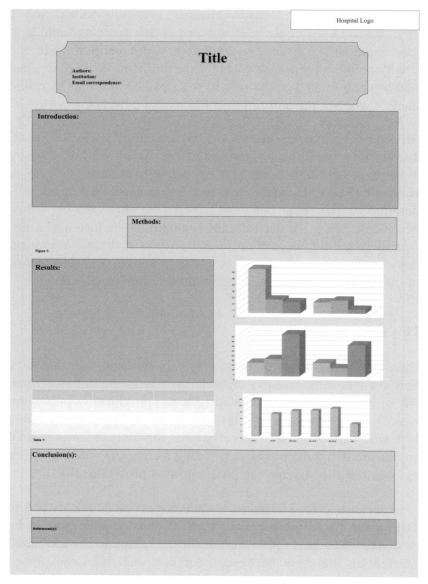

Figure 7.1   Pro forma for a poster presentation

The poster layout is important and many conferences will state the format that they want the poster to follow. It may include:

- Introduction/Background

- Objectives

- Materials and methods

- Results

- Discussion

- Conclusions

- References

- Acknowledgements.

The poster should be prepared in good time. Occasionally hospitals and universities have their own printing facilities, though it is perhaps commoner for smaller institutions to use external printing facilities. There are various choices of paper quality and weights. They may be laminated; this helps to preserve them, and adds a glossy professional finish. A roll tube or poster bag is essential to facilitate safe transportation of the poster.

When travelling abroad, it should be clarified with airlines that the poster may be allowed in the cabin. If it has to go in the hold, an electronic spare copy should be created on a 'memory stick' or CD in the event that the poster is lost.

Some conferences do not expect poster presenters to stand by their work, and allow delegates to wander around posters during the tea/coffee and lunch breaks. If this is the case, it may still be advisable at the beginning of the conference to stand by the poster; it is a good opportunity to talk informally to other delegates about the project. If the faculty is assessing the posters, a discussion of the work will be expected. The preparation for this should be similar to that described for local presentations.

Many conferences publish their posters on their website which is usually widely accessible. This is an important publication, and should provide an extra incentive to avoid spelling and grammatical errors before submitting the poster to the conference committee.

Platform presentations and lectures

A number of aspects have already been covered in this chapter, in the section entitled 'Local presentations.' Here are some more important things to remember.

Oral presentations are commonly performed by every grade of doctor. However, even for the experienced presenter it may be a daunting task.

The duration of the talk, and time allocated for questions and answers, should be readily available from the outset. Some conferences state exactly how many slides are required. It is important to ensure that the presentation software is compatible with the conference computers. One should be aware that on occasions, without any obvious reasons, videos within slides will not work.

Normally the slide show will have to be submitted in advance of the conference. It is important that on arrival at the venue, this is confirmed. As in other forms of preparations, a spare electronic copy of the presentation should be available on a 'memory stick' or CD.

It is important to practise the timing of the presentation carefully; the clock (or your watch) should be in easy view. Many mediators give speakers a 2-minute warning; this should be acknowledged (with a nod or a smile).

Sessions are generally mediated, and it is for that individual or the speaker to decide whether the floor should be open in real time or at the end of the presentation in order to answer questions. It would be ideal to have the lead auditor or senior figures available to help team working when fielding questions.

Presentations should be structured to maximise retention. Some observations have shown that this is greatest at the beginning, regresses to low levels, and then increases slightly in anticipation of the end (Ericksen 1978). Therefore planning should ensure that the main points come at a time when delegates are most attentive.

Rehearsals are vital, to assist with the content and time keeping. As always, plain and acronym-free English should be used.

Small group presentations (symposia, round table presentations)

These are essentially small scale lectures, and minor modifications may be required. When addressing the group it may be easier to sit down at the front of the room in order to engage better with the audience and maintain eye contact. There is a greater opportunity for the presentation to be interactive. The presentation style may therefore be changed, with the lecture being punctuated with questions to stimulate discussion and interaction. A flip chart, whiteboard or overhead projector may be used in preference to computerised slides to augment the presenting style. Background knowledge that is beyond reproach is more vital here, when discussions may be more fluid.

Workshop presentations

A workshop should be participative – a group that has gathered in order to share their common interest in a given subject, to extend knowledge, to improve or develop personal skills, or to solve problems by sharing common experiences and knowledge. This may be an ideal forum, therefore, to discuss implementation plans relating to an audit project. In any case the overall objective should already have been decided.

Workshop leaders or facilitators provide the format and guidelines and lead discussions so that everyone may contribute. An informal relaxed atmosphere probably works best, with seating arrangements to facilitate face-to-face discussions. Time may be set aside for introductions, where delegates are given time to get acquainted and declare their objectives. After the introductions are completed, the guidelines may be explained, the goals set and any prepared material presented to the group. The participants may subsequently be divided into smaller groups to allow all individuals to contribute. Members must be willing both to work independently and to cooperate closely. A workshop will generate more ideas than an individual working alone and will promote confidence in agreed-upon outcomes. There should therefore be provision for workshop participants to take an active part throughout. Detailed planning, including time keeping, should be meticulous.

Submission to a journal

It is rare to see clinical audits in medical journals, however this should be aspired to as they are a means of disseminating information to clinicians in the widest community.

If the whole audit group contributes as multiple authors to the paper, it is more important than ever to have a thorough plan so that the writing tasks may be divided up. Many journals now request a contributions list for the authors outlining each of their individual roles, hence it is important that all parties contribute appropriately to the paper.

Standard English should be used. The audience should be carefully considered. Clinical audits are largely going to be of interest to clinicians and members of the multidisciplinary team, and less so to scientists. Hence submitting such papers to a clinical journal that is read largely by practising clinicians is recommended.

When compiling the background, it is important to remember to include the information that is absolutely necessary to set the context of the audit and to make it easily understood. If there have been pertinent trials and/or evidence that prompted the audit, they should be carefully described and appraised in the introduction. If the audit has stemmed from a clinical observation it is useful to describe the problem in detail, because it is likely to occur elsewhere and will be helpful to the clinicians reading the article.

The materials and methods section should be the most straightforward section to write. During the audit keep a careful record should have been kept of the exact methodology, including any equipment or statistical programs used.

The 'results' section may commence with a comment on analysis and interpretation pertinent to the primary conclusion. This may be augmented by the use of tables and graphs. Statistical analyses need to be justified.

The conclusion and discussion section should deal with each of the findings in turn, commencing with the primary outcome of the audit. The importance, relevance and impact of the audit finding should be discussed, together with any consequent recommendations as a result of the audit.

When compiling the list of references, ensure that they are accurately ascribed to the text. The cited references should have been read, as occasionally a reference will have made a very different point to that attributed by another paper. The referencing style mandated by the journal should be strictly adhered to.

Appendices contain information that is not essential to the understanding of the paper, though may present facts that further clarify a point without burdening the body of the publication. This is an optional part of the paper, and is not always necessary. Each appendix should contain novel material. Some examples of material that might be put in an appendix include raw data or explanation of formulas. Figures and tables can also occasionally be found in appendices.

Which journal?

It should be remembered that most journals should have an impact factor, which is intended to factor in quality of work and readership volume. There are many well-recognised national and specialty medical journals; most of these will accept audits. In addition, there are certain clinical audit and clinical governance journals:

The International Journal for Quality in Health Care aims to make research related to quality and safety in healthcare available to a worldwide readership. The journal publishes papers in all disciplines related to the quality and safety of healthcare, including health services research, healthcare evaluation, technology assessment, health economics, utilisation review, cost containment and nursing care research, as well as clinical research related to quality of care. This peer-reviewed journal has a multidisciplinary readership and aims to include contributions from all health professions, together with quality assurance professionals, managers, politicians, social workers and researchers from health-related backgrounds. The journal also contains news of the International Society for Quality in Health Care and announcements of forthcoming courses, symposia and congresses. *The journal is* indexed by the Social Science Citation Index, Current Contents/Social and Behavioral Science, Medline (*Index Medicus*), Research Alert, Social SciSearch and Science Citation Index.

The *British Journal of Clinical Governance* was previously published as the *Journal of Clinical Effectiveness* and incorporated the *Journal of Clinical Performance and Quality Healthcare*. It *is an international journal* that aims to address the doubts, queries, triumphs and practical applications of introducing quality assurance mechanisms into the delivery of care. It takes an international stance and covers key developments worldwide, which can inform best practice in healthcare. Efficiency, effectiveness and economics are the main factors in the assessment of best practice, and all are addressed in the research, audit and evidence-based papers published.

All papers are peer-reviewed to ensure their validity and value to current debates.

The journal publishes research articles, which illustrate clear implications for practice, results-focused case studies that discuss problems and successes in clinical governance techniques, and special issues on topical themes. They cover evidence-based practice and guidelines, implementation of good practice, clinical performance indicators, audit, risk management, patient involvement and welfare, policy and strategy, and user involvement and implications. Regular sections in the journal include: North American perspectives; reviews of effectiveness from NHS Centre for Reviews and Dissemination; digests of evidence; digest of drugs from the Wolfson Unit, Newcastle; and health technology assessment executive summaries. The journal is aimed at clinical and non-clinical professionals working in a wide range of user industries, such as: clinical governance leaders; clinical directors; nursing managers/directors; general practitioners/ family doctors; practice managers; pharmaceutical companies; health insurers; academic and research institutions in medicine; and health consultants.

The journal is cited by: the British Library; *Cabell's Directory of Publishing Opportunities*; *Cambridge Scientific Abstracts*; CINAHL; EMBASE (the *Excerpta Medica* database); *Health Service Abstracts;* and SCOPUS.

Clinical Audit Today is a journal that was launched in the autumn of 2008 and is currently the only 'pure' clinical audit journal available in the UK. The journal is available online in electronic format. It is published on a quarterly basis and is keen to promote the work of all those undertaking inspiring work that is helping to reinvigorate clinical audit. The journal is aimed at clinical audit and governance staff, and practising clinicians and managers with an interest in the subject. By their own admission *Clinical Audit Today* is not intended to be a highbrow academic publication and focuses on everyday practice.

Key points

- The skills needed for presentation are generic, widely-required and essential for survival

- Presentations are also more likely to enthuse others, when compared to the simple written word

- It is vital that time is ring-fenced for clinical audit presentations

- It is good practice to allow junior doctors to travel back to their previous trust to present their project

- Be organised for all forms of presentations

- Be prepared for:

  - Local presentations

  - National and international presentations

  - Poster presentations

  - Platform presentations

  - Small group presentations

  - Workshops

  - Submission to a journal

References

Ericksen SC (1978). *The Lecture. Memo to the Faculty,* no. 60. Ann Arbor: Center for Research on Teaching and Learning, University of Michigan.

Chapter 8 Implementing change

The fundamental intervention which will prevent the project (and the theme of clinical audit in general) from becoming yet another 'tick box exercise' is the metamorphosis from project to action and from action to improved quality. This is a significant and often time-consuming undertaking, with a wide range of individuals needing to go through a period of education, changes in process and perhaps retraining.

It should be remembered that the process of clinical audit, though vitally important, provides but one single component and mechanism for the process of change. It may take clinicians a great deal of time to accept that changes in practice are needed or to decide on what implementation strategies are best. Such changes in attitude or behaviour can invariably be a slow and difficult process. Sadly, many clinical audit projects may be seen to fail when the deficiencies outlined and the recommendations suggested for improvement do not lead and translate to actual implementation.

When change is required, most commonly either to improve a level of performance or to maintain a particular standard of care, consideration must be given to a management plan for achieving this, which includes identification of potential barriers and pitfalls to change, as well as how best to combat these. Ideally, potential barriers will already have been identified at the start of the project, even before the size of any deficit is identified. Regular team meetings, interviews and conversations may have acknowledged concerns. Anonymous questionnaires may have been organised to highlight areas of anxiety.

It should be possible to outline those provisions of current practice that need improvement or modification. Perhaps, more importantly, there must be a genuine desire within a department to pursue changes which may be assumed by some as a 'risk'.

So who should be responsible for the initiation and facilitation of change and how should it be implemented? Many theories have been proposed to deal with this issue. A common scenario is that only a minority of individuals (including the auditors) understand that change is needed; there may be reticence or even fear when confronted with the problem of influencing the majority. The strategy that inevitably does not work here is that of simply asking specific, usually junior, members of the organisation to instigate the process of change unassisted.

Some barriers to implementation and some proposals

These have been discussed in Chapter 5, with regard to embarking on an audit project. It is worthwhile re-considering these issues.

Post audit, there may still be a lack of change in behaviour. This may be a consequence of:

- Lack of interest in some individuals. This may prompt a strategy where these individuals are given accountability

- Some individuals may feel that performance is good, and that therefore change is unnecessary. Perhaps the introduction of a few opinion leaders may create some influence

During the implementation process, despite the creation of high quality guidelines, the latter may not to be followed. This may be a consequence of:

- A perception amongst some individuals that they lack knowledge. This may be countered by reinforced support and education

- Denial, where perhaps the guideline is not considered reputable. Again the introduction of a few opinion leaders may be useful

Education

Audit is a very important and often underestimated tool for education in healthcare. Conversely, education is a vital tool to implement improved clinical practice. When comparing implementation tools, the medical profession probably view education with more respect than for instance guidelines and processes.

Most would agree that in most trusts, doctors' induction sessions include many irrelevancies and omit many essentials. Here, the role of clinical audit should be reinforced. The alert should also be given that new ways of working, identified through clinical audit, will be publicised in traditionally academic forums such as lectures and ward rounds.

Lecture forums may include trust-wide, divisional, directorate or departmental educational sessions. These traditionally deal with academic issues, including research and established practice. It may be innovative to include implementation items here on a cyclical (for example monthly) basis.

All doctors are familiar with the informal dissemination of knowledge (and associated 'grilling') during ward rounds. Senior clinicians may wish to inform the team of changes in practice on this stage.

Trust newsletters, reminder emails and multidisciplinary clinical governance meetings are all media which should be regularly used to spread the word.

Process and guidelines

For the purposes of practicality, there will be no distinction in this chapter between the terms 'guideline' and 'protocol'. Changes in processes are inevitably driven by the development of 'guidelines' which may be defined as 'statements of the best available clinical evidence, which help healthcare professionals with decisions about appropriate healthcare practices for specific clinical circumstances'. The aim is to improve the quality of healthcare and reduce the variation in care between healthcare professionals and different hospitals. Past research has shown that clinical practice guidelines can be effective in bringing about change and improving health outcomes (National Health and Medical Research Council 1999.)

The development of guidelines starts with a thorough literature search and critical appraisal of the information found. The resulting document should be straightforward, concise and multidisciplinary to ensure that the guidelines encompass the requirements of relevant clinicians and patient groups. They should also take into account patients' opinions, particularly on guidelines surrounding communication and quality of care. Patients have a right to their autonomy, cultural values and beliefs, which can easily be forgotten in a healthcare environment when the main focus is on 'evidence'.

Once a draft of the guideline is complete it is important that it is reviewed by all the multidisciplinary teams that have to use them. It is very common for there to be a formal process in every trust for the submission of protocols and guidelines, where each draft and the final product need to be endorsed by defined groups, and ultimately by the clinical board. Amendments will inevitably be suggested for each draft. The submission process is facilitated by the trust guideline development team. When the final draft of the guidelines is finally approved by the clinical board, it should be publicised by the trust and published on their intranet.

Simple tactics to improve the chances of implementation

It is ideal (some would say essential) to set aside a dedicated 'audit day' for the trust where a wide audience of interested parties could attend. The frequency may vary from monthly to annually, according to need. This would be the perfect well-attended forum for recommendations and implementation plans to be made by the auditors, and perhaps supported by key speakers.

Key individuals should be involved at every stage of implementation, and rapport should be established with individuals in the organisation who have the power and the gift to drive changes. Also, the organisation should be satisfied and agree with a method of implementation for instigating changes and overcoming potential barriers.

Experts who are seen as credible may be invited to deliver key lectures; they may be given time and respect by those who would otherwise be sceptical.

A multidisciplinary approach is needed to help achieve goals. Although all individuals may not agree totally with the methods of implementation, there should be some consensus for change.

The recommendations must be defined and outlined in a comprehensible fashion in order to maximise impact. Written guidelines should be distributed.

The hurdles or barriers to change should be identified and highlighted realistically, with proposed solutions. It may be prudent to plan for prospective brainstorming sessions to deal with the barriers.

The implementation process may include an element of fine detail, including the commencement date, step-by-step instructions on how tasks will be undertaken and who will ensure delivery at each step. It may be prudent to consider the necessary resources and how best they can be delivered, noting any financial constraints. The following should also be identified early:

- The groups and organisations which are affected, and hence whose support is needed for effective change to be initiated

- The method of monitoring the implementations

- The time frame for reviewing whether the actions taken have achieved their desired objective

- The method of troubleshooting (for example telephone or email availability of key individuals)

- The date for re-audit

The proposed changes in the operational process must be delineated. There should be continual assessment of quality and progress. Further changes may be needed, and additional obstacles should be identified as they arise. Therefore there should be a degree of flexibility in the process, where individuals are willing to adapt their work schedules if necessary.

Good educational strategies must be maintained post-implementation. These may include:

- Regular email updates

- Information placed on notice boards

- Information in the hospital magazine

- Regular presentations in various forums (academic or managerial)

Key points

- Education and guidelines are fundamental tools for implementation: 'project to action, and action to improved quality'

- Education: consider using traditionally academic forums such as lectures and ward rounds; doctors' inductions; newsletters; Emails; clinical governance meetings

- Guidelines: develop practical knowledge in developing guidelines and submitting them for approval by the trust

- It is ideal to identify barriers to change when embarking on the project

- It may take clinicians some time to accept changes; one should instil desire in them to implement

- There needs to be a robust management plan for implementation

- It is common for a minority of individuals to understand that change is needed, and be faced with the problem of influencing the majority

- The strategy that inevitably does not work here is that of simply asking specific, usually junior, members of the organisation to instigate the process of change unassisted

- Consider organising trust audit days to maximise uptake of implementation

- For implementation, identify early: the commencement date, groups affected, individuals responsible, method of monitoring, timeframe

- Maintain good educational strategies post-implementation

- Plan for re-auditing

References

National Health and Medical Research Council (NHMRC) (1999), *A Guide to the Development, Implementation and Evaluation of Clinical Practice Guidelines*. Available at: www.nhmrc.gov.au/publications/synopses/cp30syn. htm

National Health and Medical Research Council (NHMRC) (2000), *How to review the evidence: systematic identification and review of the scientific literature*. National Health and Medical Research Council, Canberra.

Chapter 9   Re-audit and
re-presentation

The importance of re-audit and completing the audit loop

This stage in the audit loop is simultaneously the end of the first 'cycle' and the beginning of the next one. Re-auditing should be seen as an implementation tool which has the added benefits of providing additional information about the target patients and subjects, and also facilitating improvement in clinical audit methodology.

Along with other implementation topics, the role of re-auditing often does not get much press in local audits. In contrast it should be noted that not surprisingly, national audits tend to have well-established re-audit schedules.

The best way to identify whether the recommendations made and the improvement strategy employed have had an impact on those affected, as well as on the organisation, is to carry out a re-audit. In fact this is the final and arguably most important step in completing the audit loop. It is therefore surprising that many audits fail to reach this stage and the audit loop remains uncompleted. Among the reasons cited for this inability to finish the audit process is lack of time available to those involved in the initial audit activity. It is not uncommon to find the level of interest in a topic waning, with individuals once enthusiastic about the audit process feeling less inclined to repeat their evaluation. There may be the additional perception that once again it would take them away from the clinical care of patients. By stressing the importance of quality improvement, these issues of fatigue and time constraints may be easily countered.

On consideration of the implementation strategy for improvement the clinical audit team should have set a date to re-audit. There is no set, rigid time frame for setting the date however it should be related to the time when long-term effects following implementation are most likely to be evident. It is only after meticulous analysis of the data from the original and subsequent re-audit that the group can observe the level of improvement made, and also identify the areas which remain a cause for concern. Once re-audit is performed and the audit loop is completed, two options may remain:

- If performance meets the target requirement and reflects best practice, and no new areas of concern have been highlighted, the group should plan a timetable of events that may include update meetings and presentations, and arrange a further re-audit at a subsequent date.

- If problems or areas of concern have been identified once more, the weak points in the implementation process should be reviewed and amended, and a further re-audit should be organised. If the standard is almost reached, one may simply need to tighten up the implementation and educational process.

Each NHS trust should help promote a culture of re-audit, and this should form a part of its annual auditing policy.

Rotating junior doctors

Every year or every few months, most junior doctors rotate around different departments, trusts or even regions. They may therefore not be keen to start a new audit project, as there may be the concern that they may not be available to perform a re-audit (or even present the original project). The trust, clinical audit department and senior clinicians must therefore reassure existing junior doctors that their contribution to clinical audit projects will be rewarded, even if the presentation, implementation and re-audit occurs after they move on. Recognition of involvement may take the form of a certificate sent onwards to a forwarding address. Return visits in order to present should be encouraged. New doctors who rotate into the department need to be familiar with the initial clinical audit in order to confidently re-audit. The responsibility for a rolling programme of post-implementation re-audit projects needs to be adopted by the clinical audit department, with some help and prompting from relevant clinicians and departments.

Continued relevance of criteria

The initial criteria may cease to be relevant to current practice in response to a change in local or national policy, updated research evidence or changes in patient demographics. This may occur particularly if the time set for the re-audit is too long. Criteria for the initial audit must therefore be evaluated regularly in order to maintain their relevance to current practice. A detected change in the criteria may prompt an earlier re-audit. Careful detection of changes in specific criteria for re-auditing is vital; large or numerous changes may lead to the 're-audit' slowly metamorphosing into a new audit project.

Consequences

Finally, once a re-audit has been completed, the results will influence the next steps in exactly the same fashion as the original audit project. It is recommended that the presentation is used as a vehicle to educate and remind the audience about the importance and benefit of re-auditing.

Key points

- The role of re-audit: the end of the first 'cycle' and the beginning of the next one

- Implementation tool with the added benefits of providing additional information about the target patients and subjects, and also facilitating improvement in clinical audit methodology

- Time scheduling: depends on the predicted time for implementation of the previous project recommendations and allowance for the changes to take full effect

- Rotating junior doctors: rotation may be a disincentive, therefore contribution should be encouraged and rewarded, even if the project needs to be handed over to incoming rotators; responsibility for a rolling programme of post-implementation re-audit projects needs to be adopted by the clinical audit department

- Continued relevance of criteria: initial criteria may cease to be relevant to current practice; therefore initial criteria must be evaluated regularly. A detected change in the criteria may prompt an earlier re-audit. Vigilance is needed as large or numerous changes may lead to the 're-audit' slowly metamorphosing into a new audit project

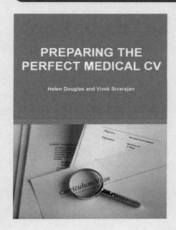

More Titles in the Progressing Your Medical Career Series

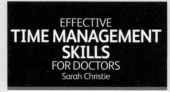

EFFECTIVE
TIME MANAGEMENT SKILLS
FOR DOCTORS
Sarah Christie

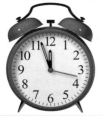

January 2009

176 pages

Paperback

ISBN 978-1-906839-08-6

£19.99

Do you find it difficult to achieve a work-life balance? Would you like to know how you can become more effective with the time you have?

With the introduction of the European Working Time Directive, which will severely limit the hours in the working week, it is moreimportant than ever that doctors improve their personal effectivenessand time management skills. This interactive book will enable youto focus on what activities are needlessly taking up your time and what steps you can take to manage your time better.

By taking the time to read through, complete the exercises and follow the advice contained within this book you will begin to:

- Understand where your time is being needlessly wasted

- Discover how to be more assertive and learn how to say 'No'

- Set yourself priorities and stick to them

- Learn how to complete tasks more efficiently

- Plan better so you can spend more time doing the things you enjoy

In recent years, with the introduction of the NHS Plan and LordDarzi's commitment to improve the quality of healthcare provision,there is a need for doctors to become more effective within their working environment. This book will offer you the chance to re-gainsome clarity on how you actually spend your time and give you the impetus to ensure you achieve the tasks and goals which are important to you.

develop
medica

More Titles in the Progressing Your Medical Career Series

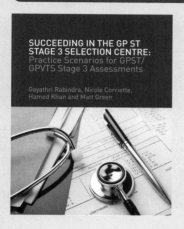

January 2009

392 pages

Paperback

ISBN 978-1-9068390-3-1

£24.99

Succeeding in the GPST Stage 3 Selection Centre is an indepth guide to help doctors fully prepare for the three different tasks that comprise this stage of the GPST Selection process. This up-to-date resource provides detailed explanation of the aims of each of the tasks you will be faced with, what they entail and the various principles that can be employed to increase your chances of success. In this book, which has been written by experts with first hand experience in this assessment, the following are addressed:

- Detailed description of the consultation, discussion and prioritisation tasks and how to approach them

- Cross reference to the person specification and markscheme - describing what the selectors are looking for, and the different ways to approach the tasks

- Ten practice scenarios for each of the three tasks to reinforce your learning together with detailed discussion of possible answers for each scenario

- Personal Perspectives - with tips from individuals who have successfully completed the selection process

- Discussion of the key concepts and terms that you will be faced with including amongst others significant event analysis and GP contracts.

Written by GPs who have first-hand experience of the process, this guide is a must have resource for any doctor serious about succeeding in their application to the GPST training scheme.

develop
medica

www.developmedica.com

A Title in the Essential Clinical Series

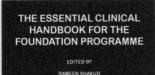

THE ESSENTIAL CLINICAL HANDBOOK FOR THE FOUNDATION PROGRAMME

EDITED BY
RAMEEN SHAKUR

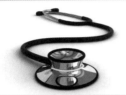

December 2009

300 pages

Paperback

ISBN 978-1-906839-09-3

Unsure of what clinical competencies you must gain to successfully complete the Foundation Programme? Unclear on how to ensure your ePortfolio is complete to enable your progression to ST training?

This up-to-date clinical handbook is aimed at current foundation doctors and clinical medical students and provides a comprehensive companion to help you in the day-to-day management of patients on the ward. Together with this it is the first handbook to also outline clearly how to gain the core clinical competencies required for successful completion of the Foundation Programme. Written by doctors for doctors this comprehensive handbook explains how to successfully manage all of the common cases you will face during the Foundation Programme and:

- Introduces the Foundation Programme and what is expected of a new doctor especially with the introduction of Modernising Medical Careers

- Illustrates clearly the best way to manage, step-by-step, over 150 commonly encountered clinical diseases, including NICE guidelines to ensure a gold standard of clinical care is achieved.

- Describes how to successfully gain the core clinical competencies within Medicine and Surgery including an extensive list of differentials and conditions explained

- Explores the various radiology images you will encounter and how to interpret them

- Tells you how to succeed in the assessment methods used including DOP's, Mini-CEX's and CBD's.

- Has step by step diagrammatic guide to doing common clinical procedures competently and safely.

- Outlines how to ensure your ePortfolio is maintained properly to ensure successful completion of the Foundation Programme.

- Provides tips and advice on how to start preparing now to ensure you are fully prepared and have the competitive edge for your CMT/ST Application.

The introduction of the ePortfolio as part of the Foundation Programme has paved the way for foundation doctors to take charge of their own learning and portfolio. Through following the expert guidance laid down in this handbook you will give yourself the best possible chance of progressing successfully through to CMT/ST training.

develop
medica

www.developmedica.com